ARTHRITIS, RHEUMATISM
AND PSORIASIS

Books by the Same Author

Arthritis, Rheumatism and Psoriasis

Jan de Vries

By Appointment Only series

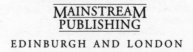

MAINSTREAM
PUBLISHING

EDINBURGH AND LONDON

First published in Great Britain in 1986 by
MAINSTREAM PUBLISHING COMPANY
(Edinburgh) Ltd
7 Albany Street
Edinburgh EH1 3UG

Reprinted 1987, 1989 1991, 1992,
1994, 1997, 2003

ISBN 1 84018 558 9

A catalogue record for this book is available
from the British Library

Typeset in Century Old Style
Printed and bound in Great Britain by
Cox & Wyman Ltd

Contents

Foreword

SOME YEARS AGO, after the birth of my fifth child, and having left the maternity hospital a couple of days after the birth, I was showing off my state of fitness to my family by hanging out the washing. I became aware of some discomfort in my neck, which later developed into the most severe pain I have ever experienced. A hormone called Relaxin, produced by the body to facilitate childbirth and still circulating in my system, had helped to dislocate the fifth cervical vertebra in my neck. The only way to get me out of bed was for my husband to cup his hands behind my neck and give me a very painful lift. The night before I was to be admitted to hospital, as this painful manoeuvre took place, there was a loud report from my neck and an immediate relief of pain. I had just experienced my first neck adjustment, albeit at the hands of a very unskilled manipulator.

From this time I suffered bouts of neck pain, accompanied by tingling in my fingers and, worst of all, dizziness and unsteadiness of gait. Patients are not inspired with confidence by the sight of their doctor staggering about the consulting room! Wearing my surgical collar prolonged my consulting time, as I had to explain about my disability to each patient. Massage, traction and heat treatment all failed to relieve my problem.

A friend showed great concern for my predicament and, despite my reluctance and scepticism, persuaded me to go with her to Troon to consult the now famous 'Healing Dutchman'. Meeting Jan de Vries opened new horizons. After two treatments with acupuncture and neck adjustment, and many doses of Araniforce, my neck problem disappeared. Soon I was sending many of my own patients with spinal problems on the road to Troon.

Jan and I have done a lot of work together over the past two years. I am grateful for the opportunity of working with and learning from him. This has been of great benefit to myself and to my own patients with special problems.

This book, Jan's fourth, is about arthritis. It describes the alternative approach to treatment of this crippling disease in all its forms. Rheumatoid arthritis is one of the most painful and debilitating diseases to afflict mankind. It can strike at any age and causes much misery, not only to the victim but to his or her whole family. Of my 2,500 patients I have twenty-three cases, so it is not an uncommon illness. Osteoarthritis in all its manifestations can also be very disabling and it is one of the most common ailments we GPs have to deal with.

One of my patients had been housebound with rheumatoid arthritis as long as I had known her and, despite having been treated with a cornucopia of medicines, still suffered from large weeping nodules in many joints, as well as the usual pain and stiffness. After treatment from Jan she is now able to go shopping and last year even visited her daughter in America.

My brother, also a GP, developed rheumatoid arthritis three years ago. The two drugs initially used to treat him have now been removed from the drug list by the Committee for Safety of Drugs. Neither had relieved his pain and stiffness anyway. I eventually persuaded him to see Jan. After his initial doubt about taking Jan's 'liquidised grass', as he cynically referred to the medication, he had a noticeable improvement in his joints within a short period. He is now very happy to continue taking the same 'liquidised grass' and, like myself, he refers a number of his patients for treatment by the alternative methods. Many people with different types of arthritis have benefited from Jan's dietary advice, acupuncture and medication. What I like about this method of treatment is that the medication not only is effective, but also causes no hepato cellular damage, no bone marrow, depression and no gastric upset, side-effects unfortunately seen all too often with modern drug treatment.

No one yet knows all the answers about the cause of this terrible affliction. However, Jan has found more answers than most. This man, with his vast knowledge, has given arthritic sufferers much comfort and has also given orthodox practitioners much food for thought.

Dr Sarah T.P. Marr, MB, ChB, 1986

1

Rheumatoid Arthritis

SEVERAL YEARS AGO, an attractive lady in her middle forties, whom I had known for at least fifteen years, came to see me. I remembered her visiting our residential clinic along with her husband for a course of general treatment. At that time they were a basically healthy couple with nothing wrong with them. The lived a careful life in that they neither smoked nor drank and both followed a well-balanced diet.

I had not seen her for a number of years and I noticed that her once beautiful hands and fingers had turned into gnarled, swollen claws and enlarged, twisted knuckles. The rest of her body had also stiffened and twisted. I wondered how her health had been allowed to deteriorate to such an extent and how rheumatoid arthritis could have taken such a grip. It is because of these so far unanswered questions that I have hundreds of other patients visiting our clinic every week.

Though I paint a terrible picture here, such a sight is all too familiar when we look around us. Many people are stricken with prolonged periods of severe pain, which makes moving, sitting and sleeping difficult. The only relief is some pain-killing drug which after a while has a less and less helpful effect. Cortisone is often prescribed, but again this does not produce a cure. Once such treatment has commenced, it is generally necessary for life.

I took a long time to interview this particular lady, for the simple reason that she was desperate for help and prepared to co-operate fully, which in cases of arthritis is very necessary. Where did she go wrong in her lifestyle? Was there maybe a connection with the 'change of life' which she had just started? Or were there other reasons?

Ladies approaching middle age and the inevitable change of life very often suffer from hormone irregularities and the resulting imbalance could in some cases be a cause of this problem.

I discussed the balance of her diet with my patient and felt that there were certain vitamin, mineral and trace element deficiencies. Another factor which did not help, however, was that her place of work had concrete flooring. The energy flow which should help her is cut off by the wearing of rubber-soled shows and by concrete floors.

The smallest things can influence patients who are prone to any kind of arthritis. Several of those known to us will be discussed in this book. I have seen many patients over the years and have also been able to help many of them. I felt that this lady was not beyond help and we immediately decided on a programme containing a well-balanced diet, a few natural remedies and some acupuncture treatment. I was convinced that after a while she would begin to experience some relief. I have often witnessed in the past that these swollen fingers and enlarged knuckles will reduce in size if the body is steered in the right direction.

Millions of pounds have been spent by clinics and research associations, but seemingly to little avail because a definite cure for rheumatism and arthritis has still not been found. In the field of alternative medicine, though, there is at last a strong possibility of a breakthrough. For the past hundred years or more the application of herbal and homoeopathic therapies have produced remarkable results. It is, therefore, well worth anyone suffering from these and related problems seriously considering alternative therapy.

It is now generally accepted, too, that although some people may inherit tendencies towards certain ailments from their forebears, incorrect diet greatly contributes towards producing illnesses like arthritis and rheumatism. Our diet should be absolutely natural and acid-forming foods, in particular pork and processed meats, should be excluded. A correction of our diet, combined with treatment by herbal and homoeopathic remedies can provide great relief from these crippling diseases which, especially in the UK, are so much on the increase.

Which influences on our bodies lead to the development of these conditions? Well, an important one is stress, which is everything and anything that threatens or damages us – fear, a heavy workload, our diet. In the stressful world we live in, there are many factors which affect us. Some stress, however, is avoidable, as we can discipline ourselves to stop smoking, for example. It is of the utmost importance that we learn to meet stress and tackle it. Physically, we must learn to keep putting back what we take out of our bodies. Our nutrition must therefore be very good.

At the base of the brain there is a tiny gland called the pituitary. At any sign of stress this gland releases a hormone which sounds the alarm. The hormone travels in the blood until it reaches two small glands that sit on our kidneys in the middle of the back, the adrenals. When the adrenal glands pick up this hormone, they too release their own hormones. The chief of these is called cortisol (which we also know as cortisone).

Messages also reach the adrenals from the nervous system and the hormone adrenaline is released. The presence of these adrenal hormones in the blood tells the whole body that it is under threat.

The body's reaction is quite dramatic: sugar reserves pour into the blood for immediate fuel; proteins and fats are broken down to make more energy; calcium is taken from our bones to be used by nerve and muscle; pain, stiffness and inflammation miraculously disappear; blood pressure rises so that oxygen, sugar and calcium travel more quickly to the tissues. This stress reaction is highly protective. Normally the threat ends and the above reactions are reversed. Proteins are built up again and the cells repaired; calcium is put back into our bones; blood pressure drops to normal and all our familiar aches and pains reappear. The body's reserves will have been spent and even more nutrients will be needed for repairs. More vitamins, minerals, protein, fats and carbohydrates will be needed than usual.

The adrenals produce cortisol from the hormone

deoxycortisol (DOC for short). DOC itself has a remarkable action. It helps the body fight infection and damage by setting up inflammation around bacteria or toxins and walling them off, as in boils for example. Swelling, pain and fever may result, but the body will have been protected. Normally, sufficient DOC will be converted to cortisol to remove the pain and swelling once the intruder has been dealt with.

When the diet does not supply the vitamins needed by the enzymes that make and balance these hormones, the DOC may fail to be converted and the area of pain and swelling may become permanent and collect calcium. Cortisone treatment is not the easy solution. This inhibits our own DOC production, thus lowering resistance. Our bones become further demineralised and other mineral reactions cause water retention (moon face). The constant robbing of proteins may eat away our stomach cells and give us ulcers.

The whole vitamin spectrum must be used when nutrition has broken down so severely. Aspects of our diets must change. When we eat sugar our blood sugar level rises quickly and we feel full of energy, which is why we like it. Another gland, the pancreas, is alerted and insulin is released to take the sugar and store it. When we eat sugar frequently our pancreas becomes trigger-happy and takes out too much at a time. We then develop low blood sugar, or hypoglycaemia. The adrenals are alerted and we go into stress reaction. Calcium is taken from our bones. So when we eat sugar we can cause 'holes' in our bones, not just in our teeth.

When our nutrition is inadequate at this point, or when the stress situation does not come to an end, our body will come under further threat. By robbing Peter to pay Paul, it will do the best it can for as long as it can, but sooner or later we will find that we have no more reserves and that we make no more adrenal hormones. In other words, we have no further resistance. Disease is the result.

The removal of calcium from the bones when under stress is clearly one feature of the arthritic process. Normally, calcium moves continuously between blood and bone to maintain a balance. A hormone from the parathyroid glands in the neck takes calcium from the bones when the blood level drops. Calcitonin, a hormone from the thyroid gland, encourages calcium back to the bone. Vitamins are needed for us to absorb calcium from our food and also to help the bone to mineralise.

The balance of calcium in the body is very delicate. If the blood level drops, our muscles go into spasms and convulsions. If our bones are continuously leached, they may bend or break. If blood calcium stays high, as in stress, then calcium may be deposited in arteries, tissues, muscles and joints. This tendency appears to be caused by prolonged stress without adequate nutrition, a parathyroid imbalance or vitamin deficiency.

Few of us realise that we are addicted to salt. Salt is a stimulant. It hits the adrenals and we go into stress reaction. Most of us eat ten times too much salt in a day because we like the 'high'.

The blood is naturally 80 per cent alkaline. The alkaline-forming foods are mainly fruit and vegetables, yoghurt and seeds. If we eat an all-acid meal, such as an egg on toast with coffee, we use up calcium and other minerals in our body's effort to restore the alkaline balance. It is difficult to heal arthritis in an acid body. Our intake therefore should be 80 per cent alkaline and 20 per cent acid.

Calcium must be added to the diet during the healing programme. The bones will only remineralise when there is sufficient calcium in the diet. Calcium enters into solution in an acid medium and is precipitated and deposited in an alkaline medium. This simple but profound statement provides the key to unlock the mystery of arthritis.

To reverse this process – one of solubility – we must employ a secondary agent. This agent is potassium.

Nowadays we can realise why arthritis and related diseases occur so frequently. We only need to look at the 'anti-sources' of potassium, which form such a regular part of our diet and lifestyle, for example alcohol, coffee, laxatives, salt, sugar and stress. Good sources of potassium on the other hand are: potatoes, bananas, dates, figs, molasses, cider-vinegar, apricots and raisins. We should eat plenty of these foods.

In every type of arthritis, the diet of the patient has to be altered from a poor sub-nutritive diet to an energy-producing one particularly rich in potassium. Potassium deficiency can produce rapid calcification of the arteries, muscles and joints. A diet low in potassium causes types of arthritis which are preceded by rheumatic disorders – aching muscles first, and fixed joints afterwards. Diet, therefore, is very important.

I advise all arthritis patients and patients suffering from arthritis-related diseases never to eat any of the following: pork, sausages, bacon, ham, gammon, white flour, white sugar, oranges, lemons, grapefruit, tomatoes, vinegar, mayonnaise, rhubarb, butter, cream and spices. It is also advisable to reduce the intake of tea and coffee, and salt should be used sparingly. Better still, use a good sea salt like A.Vogel's Herbamare.

Rheumatic or arthritic sufferers should eat lots of fresh vegetables, either raw or cooked, a salad every say, plenty of fruit, nuts, honey, cottage cheese, brown rice and natural yoghurt.

To make sure that our potassium intake is sufficient, I advise frequently that Joint Mobility Factors tablets are taken. To regulate the most important gland, the thyroid, kelp is ideal. Again this is available in tablet form and I usually recommend A.Vogel Kelp tablets from the Bioforce range of herbal products.

I have designed a programme for people suffering from arthritis and related diseases in which both the above-mentioned products feature. Also included in this programme is the herbal remedy Knotgrass Complex which was formulated by Alfred Vogel many years ago. This remedy contains herbs which are traditional cleansers and healers, and these are used to bring body, mind and emotions back into healing alignment. Knotgrass Complex gives amazing results. After only a few weeks, swelling which might have affected several parts of the body, is reduced or disappears. It contains extracts of knotgrass, musk yarrow, birch, golden rod, horsetail, silverweed, nettle and peppermint. This wonderful remedy should be taken with a cup of Golden Grass tea, which is a composition of several dried herbs.

I also frequently recommend that about 1,000 to 2,000 mg of vitamin C should be taken daily and, if at all possible, plenty of rest and sunshine.

The question remains: can rheumatism and

arthritis be successfully treat at home? The answer must be affirmative and a good start may be achieved if the above instructions are adhered to.

It is wonderful to see that with even a little help the human body may benefit. I often advise taking some potato juice every morning. Take a large unpeeled potato, wash it well, grate it and press the juice out of it with a spoon. This is a wonderful remedy to restore the acid and alkaline balance in the human body. It is also a very effective antidote for uric acid conditions. Together with the potato juice some simple mustard seeds may be chewed. I have many testimonials on file which show that rheumatic or arthritic problems can be relieved or solved by this simple and inexpensive method.

It is important to remember that arthritis is not in truth a disease in itself, but that it is produced by other diseases or body malfunctions. It is found in the connective tissue and so causes inflammation in one or more joints and the related tissues. The commonly used term 'arthritis' covers a multitude of sins. The inflammation which demonstrates itself as heat, swelling, redness and pain is damaging to the tissue. It is severely crippling, but it does not kill.

Looking back in history, we realise that arthritis is a very old and chronic disease. Archaeologists have come across reptile fossils from thousands of years back where evidence of arthritic conditions was present. Indications of arthritis in the spine have been found in the bones of our ancestors and some Egyptian mummies carry signs of arthritis. Many of us have recollections of grandparents struggling with this most painful and crippling disease.

Although it is said that the cause of rheumatoid arthritis is not known, a relation to infection, allergy, metabolic disorder or endocrine problem is postulated. The disease is more common in temperate climates. Seventy-five per cent of the patients are female and in 80 per cent of all cases there is an onset before the age of forty. Rheumatoid arthritis is severely disabling and progressive: long and perseverant treatment is needed. A good understanding between the patient and the practitioner is therefore imperative.

I remember the case of a lady from the Midlands who consulted me. She was in an advanced rheumatic condition and had been subjected to various different forms of treatment by her rheumatologist. Fortunately, between them they had managed to keep her out of a wheelchair, but she was severely handicapped. I tried to make her realise the importance of diet and had to stress that she cut out all acid and high protein foods. I also explained the importance of alleviating her chronic constipation. Alfred Vogel often stated in his lectures that the acid/alkaline balance is extremely important to arthritic patients, whereas the protein/carbohydrate balance needs to be looked at to ease constipation problems.

Carbohydrates burn up like wood in the fire. We know that if we burn wood, we are left with dust and ashes. High protein foods, like meat and other products, burn up like coal in the fire and we know what happens when coal burns. It burns out and we are left with stones and cinders.

I remember an old doctor telling me once that most diseases stem from the bowels and explaining the importance of a regular motion every morning – hence the reason that doctors used to advise their patients to take castor oil in order to move the bowels regularly.

I managed to convince this lady patient of the importance of regular bowel movement and I recommended some herbal remedies to her. As she was very anaemic, which is very often the case with arthritic patients, I told her to eat plenty of fresh green vegetables. Twice a week she should take a dessert of four dried pears soaked overnight in a red, sweet wine or grape juice. This enriches the blood. She should also regularly take two eggs beaten with some grape juice. On top of this I gave her some general dietary advice. To my surprise I received a letter from her hospital consultant some months later. He was intrigued by my approach to this patient, who was rapidly improving.

I am reminded of a young medical student who set out to test me. He asked me to tell him the early symptoms of arthritis. I said that there were a variety of ways in which this could manifest itself and listed some:

a general feeling of weakness;

inability to feel connections between muscle and joints when lifting or pulling;

inability to achieve as much physically as we used to;

extreme fatigue, even on rising in the morning; feelings of sometimes not being able to put our feet properly on the ground;

pains in the lower back, knees or other joints;

a very stiff feeling when kneeling and getting up again;

tingling sensations in fingertips and hands;

pains and stiffening of joints;

tender feelings and swellings in one or more joints;

unexplained weight loss, sometimes quite severe;

a feeling that the joints do not move as they are supposed to.

The student looked at me and said that I was quite right. He had experienced several of these symptoms during the past year. He was also curious to know if unpleasant past emotional experiences could have played a part, to which I answered in the affirmative. Traumatic experiences can influence the condition of people suffering from arthritis or related diseases. He confided in me that he had been through a difficult period, due to financial hardship which had jeopardised his studies. He had also broken off his relationship with his girlfriend. Thereafter he had discovered signs of eczema. He was told that he was suffering from several allergies and that his dietary habits were appalling. All these things together formed a perfect breeding ground for a real rheumatoid arthritic condition.

During our talk I pointed out how many individuals were attacked by one form of arthritis or another. In his case, however, it was not surprising that he had reached the state that he was in, considering the contributory factors. He is now a happy man and free from all his previous problems.

Experiences of this kind encourage me to help the thousands of arthritic patients I have met over the years. Despite expensive and extensive research no cure has yet been discovered for rheumatic complaints and therefore it would be wise to look to the more simple forms of treatment. The secret of success in treating an arthritic patient is to understand the cause. Once a causative picture is formed, the treatment may be decided on.

I recall a 20-year-old girl who had tremendous problems with her hands. She was diagnosed by a rheumatologist to be suffering from rheumatoid arthritis and had gone through several forms of treatment. Her skin was in a deplorable state and felt that she would benefit from a good cleansing programme. She told me that she was very sleepy in the morning and needed a few hours before waking up properly. She always felt tired and had considerable problems in connection with her bowel movements. She had almost developed an inferiority complex about her skin problems.

As she did not lack intelligence, she realised that in order to achieve results she needed to co-operate fully. I impressed on her that unless she was willing to follow a good cleansing diet, there would be no healing for her and I quoted a saying of Johann Schroth:

> Without battle – no victory.
> Without self-denial – no satisfaction.
> Without cleansing – no healing.

I told her to hang this quotation above her bed and to remember that this piece of old wisdom was of great importance to her. She attended the clinic fortnightly and I reminded her regularly that without cleansing she could not expect healing. With a smile she promised that she was doing everything she was told. She was delighted when after six months of treatment the results started to become noticeable and she became a fervent swimmer, enjoying life to the full.

I told this girl that the famous Prof. Dr Christiaan Barnard, the surgeon who performed the first heart transplant operation, suffered for years from rheumatism. In an interview he declared that because of a good cleansing, raw, wholefood diet he had been able to keep his symptoms in check. As a result of combating his allergies he had ended up as a much happier man. He said how encouraging it was that he could speak of almost total healing.

It is said that more than eight million people in this country alone are afflicted with arthritis of one form or another. Although rheumatism and arthritis are surrounded by many myths, there is a key to help solve these problems as long as everyone is considered as an individual. The majority of sufferers of arthritis and related diseases do react very well to the simple dietary instructions which I have already mentioned. For more serious cases, however, I advise that a stricter diet be adhered to.

The broad outlines of this dietary regime are as follows:

Preparatory five-day cleansing programme
Breakfast: fresh or stewed fruit
Lunch: a salad or vegetable soup; fresh fruit
Supper: cooked fresh vegetables and salad; fresh fruit

Exclude: Potatoes, tomatoes, oranges and bananas
Only drink herbal teas, bottled water or diluted fresh fruit juices.
After five days start on the main diet. A choice can be made from items listed under each section.

Breakfast
Stewed or fresh fruit (excluding oranges)
Cereal, such as muesli or Jordan's Original Crunchy (if required, sweetened with molasses), moistened with water, soya milk, apple juice or date juice.
Rye crispbread, brown rice or barley with soya sauce.

Lunch
A salad containing any raw vegetable except tomatoes. A celery-based salad is especially good, to which grated apple and sprouting seeds may be added.

Blended vegetable soup or soup from vegetable stock cubes available from health food shops.

Rye crispbread.

Jacket potato.

Any whole grain, such as barley, rice millet, or buckwheat, as long as no polished grains are used.

Dinner

Fresh sea fish – not more than four times per week.

Shellfish – only once a week.

Lamb – only once a week.

Pulses such as aduki beans, kidney beans or haricot beans; lentils or chickpeas; up to three times a week.

Tofu – not more than three times per week.

At least two meals per week should consist of brown rice and sautéed vegetables only.

Cooked vegetables and bean sprouts – only fresh produce is to be used.

Potatoes, brown rice, millet, barley or rice.

Beverages

China or Earl Grey tea without milk or sugar.

Any fresh fruit juices (except orange juice). Apple juice is especially recommended.

Mineral water.

Herbal teas such as chamomile, juniper berry or elderflower.

Seasonings

Salads may be dressed with lemon juice, olive oil or cider vinegar.

For cooking use olive oil, sunflower oil, soya oil or pure vegetable oil margarines.

Garlic is excellent, but generally herbs should be used sparingly.

Sea salt should also be used minimally, as well as soya sauce.

For sweetening, honey, molasses or brown sugar may be used.

Food to be avoided

Chocolate, cheese, citrus fruit, beef, pork, poultry, eggs, coffee, red wine, sherry, port, excess alcohol, malt vinegar, bread, any flour products such as cakes, biscuits, buns, pasta, etc., cordials, fizzy drinks, white sugar, common salt, any processed foods, smoked foods and pickled foods.

Supplements

Because of the dietary restrictions certain supplements are advised and mostly I recommend Alfred Vogel's preparations. Take the following supplements daily:

2 cod liver oil capsules

500 mg calcium pantothenate

2,000 mg vitamin C

200 i.u. vitamin E

3 vitamin B12 capsules

4 Kelp tablets

I have also introduced Sea-tone to this programme, which has a green-lipped mussel extract.

In the late 1970s a lady from a neighbouring town came to see me. She suffered from stiffening of the joints and various other complaints related to rheumatoid arthritis. I started by advising her on dietary requirements and recommended some homoeopathic remedies. Although she showed some improvement, the results were not exceptional. On one of her subsequent visits she brought a newspaper article with her, which her daughter had sent her from Australia.

The article concerned a product which was extracted from the New Zealand green-lipped mussel, whose Latin name is *Perna canaliculus*. The extract was obtained from the gonads or sex glands of the green-lipped mussel and freeze-dried. According to this article many arthritic and rheumatic people had benefited from this product.

Needless to say, I started making inquiries, but was unable to get information anywhere in Britain. I decided to contact the manufacturers named in the article, MacFarlane Laboratories in New Zealand, direct, as they were reported to have meticulously researched the results obtained by their product. They were kind enough to send me some capsules, which I gave to several of my patients with their full knowledge and approval. Most of them seemed to benefit more or less immediately from these capsules, which obviously delighted me and I decided to do some further tests.

From information received I learned that of the many kinds of shellfish, the New Zealand green-lipped mussel in particular contained important elements beneficial to arthritic patients. They are cultivated in seawater basins, from which the contents are systematically checked and controlled. Because treatments in our clinic are based on natural foods and homoeopathic principles, in which we have included amongst others hydrotherapy, osteopathy and naturopathy, I was very interested.

After about three months I was able to tell this lady patient that, thanks to the newspaper article she had brought to me, this new remedy had been introduced into our clinic. Through this policy, not only she, but any other arthritic patients now were given an opportunity to realise an improvement in their health. I tried to set up a programme with the co-operation of some of the many arthritic patients who attended our clinic – a programme combining diet, manipulation, physiotherapy and oral medication in the form of homoeopathic or herbal remedies. There is no doubt that arthritis patients do benefit from such a programme – based on achieving the correct acid/alkaline balance and including the green-lipped mussel extract as well as several natural remedies from Alfred Vogel.

After the green-lipped mussel extract had become better known in Britain, I was informed that a research programme was being set up by two friends and colleagues of mine, the doctors Sheila and Robin Gibson, who practise at the Homoeopathic Hospital in Glasgow. Together with several of their colleagues they aimed to prove that this product lived up to its, by now, high expectations. The characteristic properties of the New Zealand green-lipped mussel had already been extensively researched and the outcome of these tests in Glasgow underlined previous findings.

I was also very pleased with the detailed report I received on tests which had taken place at a health clinic in the Scottish Highlands. Patients participating in this test programme were prescribed 250 mg of Sea-tone per day. The duration of the tests was six months and involved 29 rheumatic arthritic patients and 66 patients suffering from osteoarthritis, which meant a mixture of painful backs, fibrositis, sciatica and other complaints. The average age of the rheumatic arthritic patients was 53.4 years, while that of the osteoarthritic patients was 67.1 years. The patients varied in age from 45 to 88 years.

It was interesting that from 29 rheumatoid arthritis patients (28 ladies and one gentleman), 7 patients showed some signs of improvement and the remaining 22 patients reported good results. After having followed the programme for two to three weeks, most patients started to notice an improvement. It must be realised, however, that as these patients were under strict supervision, speedier results were obtained than if this programme were followed at home. Obviously, without clinical supervision one tends to be slightly less strict with the diet.

The osteoarthritis group (58 ladies and 8 gentlemen) generally experienced good results. Of the 66 patients 52 reported good progress and 14 extremely good results. Some of these patients were even able to go for walks in the hilly surroundings of the clinic.

Detailed reports of all these tests were produced – proving that by using Sea-tone speedy results may be obtained – and published in the medical press.

One of our favourite Samoyed dogs started to move about stiffly. She was about ten years old, and after I had given her green-lipped mussel extract for a short period, I could hardly believe my eyes when

I saw her chase a rabbit again in the woods at the back of our clinic. I was delighted to see how much more supple and energetic she had become again.

Before I moved to Scotland I was connected with a residential health clinic based on natural medicine. In this clinic we had many rheumatic patients and I often wonder, had we been aware at the time of the beneficial properties of the green-lipped mussel extract, whether we would have been able to achieve more worthwhile results with many of those patients.

Nowadays, in the medical world, steroids and anti-inflammatory drugs are used in the first instance for treatment of rheumatic patients, followed by gold injections. Even though these medicines seem to produce speedy relief, this does not appear to last. Alternative remedies are often equally effective but are unfortunately underrated by many in the medical profession. Patients find it confusing that the mussel extract is often ignored by their own doctors and specialists, though I have noticed that this is changing gradually. No side effects have been discovered during the many extensive research programmes which have taken place with the mussel extract.

Whilst writing this book I received a letter written by an elderly patient, who reminded me that it had been approximately seven months since he had come to consult me about his rheumatism. He wrote about his incredible progress and mentioned he was again able to bend his head back and see the ceiling above him. His wife, having witnessed his improved condition, reminded him that this would be one of the many jobs round the house he would soon be able to undertake once more. He told me that he always kept a small amount of the mussel extract in reserve and felt that if for any reason he deviated from the prescribed diet, he could soon rectify any short-term damage.

I am very often asked the question, 'How long will it take for me to lead a normal life again, if ever?' The answer is always the same: 'It varies from one person to another.' Full co-operation is necessary and we also have to learn to understand how to rebuild our immune system, to recognise our natural enemies and how to influence our own body cells. Don't let us ever forget that our immune system draws its energy from three sources, namely: food, water and air. We all know that every single one of these three sources is under attack in this day and age.

We have a large variety of processed and semi-processed foods, called convenience foods, with all their colourings and additives, yet the fibre and roughage which are so necessary for our health are often omitted. The water we drink is tampered with in many ways, not least by the fluoridation process in many parts of Britain. The air we breathe is badly polluted and here I only need to mention the exhaust fumes.

Can we then still combat disease today? The answer is a definite 'Yes' – if we concentrate on all the possibilities left to rebuild our immune system. It is therefore so important in today's civilisation that this system is nourished with energy-giving foods.

In this book, energy will be mentioned on more than one occasion, stressing the importance of energy to the human body. A number of years ago I was privileged to be asked to speak at a conference in Cologne, Germany. Thousands of people were gathered there and at the end of the conference I was invited to join a subcommittee. We were asked to compose a statement to remind governments the world over of their responsibility to the health of the world's population in relation to energy. In the last paragraph of our statement we stipulated that to promote the health of the populace the right source of energy should be used. Extreme care should be taken with those forms of energy which could also be applied for military and armaments purposes.

One of our committee members specifically asked that we stress the importance that everyone responsible for human rights and health should be made aware of the dangers of choosing the wrong kind of energy. When the meeting had finished I was pleased to be able to talk further with this gentleman, whose attitude had intrigued me. He was introduced to me as Prof. Schaumberg from Brazil. I learned that he had been involved in the development of nuclear weapons and was fully aware of the dangers we had been discussing. He insisted, however,, that there is still much ignorance and we really know little as yet about energy. According to him, we are still only scraping the surface of it. Prof. Schaumberg made it quite clear that although energy is given to us in many forms, we should adhere to the simple knowledge to live our lives as naturally as possible, in order to maintain our health.

If we can do nothing more, let us pay extra care and attention to the three forms of energy from which we receive life: food, water and air. Let us try to keep these life-giving sources as unspoilt and as pure as possible.

2

Osteoarthritis

IT NEVER CEASES to amaze me how doctors and practitioners tend to lose sight of the fact that each patient deserves to be treated as an individual. If any measure of success is to be achieved, the patient must be treated and not the disease. If often surprises me when I see patients who have been diagnosed by rheumatologists in hospital that they don't even know whether they have rheumatoid arthritis or osteoarthritis. These two kinds of arthritis are very often confused. Before treating the patient, the practitioner has to study that person and sometimes has to be a bit of a detective to discover the background of the problems. In the process of labelling the patient and advising on suitable treatment, the patient must always remain an individual.

Arthritis in general can be caused by many features. By delving into the background of the patient we discover a large percentage of cases where the cause is not due to dietary imbalance or traumatic experiences. Very often emotional strain may be at the root of it, such as an unhappy marriage, career disappointments, daily frustration, worry, fear and other comparable problems. Although there is a large quantity of literature about rheumatoid arthritis, osteoarthritis and related diseases, many questions still remain unanswered. How often do we hear the statement: 'We don't really know what arthritis is or, rather, why some people are more susceptible to it than others, therefore there is no effective cure.'

Sometimes it is said that osteoarthritis is a form of menopausal syndrome, caused by endocrine disturbance, ageing, deficiencies or a traumatic degenerative joints disease. It can, however, be very wearying and painful, especially when hard bony swellings have formed.

An experiment at the Royal Free Hospital in London some years ago gave us a very clear picture of how different kinds of arthritis can be treated by raw food diets as advocated by Dr Bircher-Benner. It was interesting that particularly infectious arthritis patients made tremendous improvement. The progress of the patients undergoing this programme was filmed and after several weeks one of the patients was visited by her daughter, who could not believe that she was looking at the same person, as the improvement was so dramatic. This experiment showed that much can be done with a specially developed diet for arthritis in combination with herbal and homoeopathic medication.

Selenium has been administered to arthritic patients, who seem to have reacted very well to it. Even if taken in minute quantities, severely handicapped patients have shown overall improvement. Due to artificial manuring and fertilising, the soil has become deficient in this mineral. As a result, the food grown in this soil also displays the same deficiencies. Therefore selenium, as well as some trace minerals, when added to the diet of an osteoarthritic person may be very beneficial. Very often such simple measures can prove effective.

In one of my earlier books, *Traditional Home and Herbal Remedies*, I have given several old 'folk' remedies, like the cod liver oil cure, as well as other cures and poultices which may be helpful to arthritic people.

On one occasion, while shopping in one of the main shopping centres, I met a lady who had visited my clinic many years previously. She looked fit and well, going about her business as if she never had suffered from arthritis in her life. I wished I had taken her picture when she arrived in my clinic so many years ago, when she was hardly able to walk. She came with the message that she had been diagnosed as suffering from osteoarthritis. After examining her I had to tell her that with the treatment I was going to suggest, her symptoms would become much more bothersome and painful before there would be any improvement. We discussed the whole background of the illness and I explained the treatment to her. Indeed, she did get considerably worse. When her appointment for her sixth treatment was due, her husband had to carry her in because she could not walk. We continued the treatment and she started to improve slightly, but she was very depressed.

I had to encourage her constantly and told her to keep up the good work, because it would pay off eventually. At one stage, when she was about to give up, I remember telling her that within three months she would be so much better. This all happened years ago and there I saw her, fit and well, happily serving behind the counter of her shop. She told many people of her experiences and stressed the point that her perseverance had been rewarded.

While writing about this lady in the shopping centre, I am reminded of another time when I was out to do some messages. A gentleman spoke to me and asked if I would say hello to his wife who was across the road. I crossed the road with him and greeted his wife, who was sitting in a wheelchair, completely crippled. With tears in her eyes she spoke to me and said: 'I wished, doctor, that I had listened to you, because if I had, I would not now be sitting in this chair.' I remembered that she had had several treatments and had noticed some improvement. She was mobile and felt that the improvement would continue even if the treatment was stopped. The actual words used were: 'I think we can call it a day.' I told her that whatever she did, she should continue the treatment until she had completely recovered. She did not pay any heed to the dietary advice I had given her, nor to any other counsel. She now told me that her condition had steadily deteriorated and eventually she had to be pushed around in the wheelchair. More is the pity, because if she had continued with the treatment, she would have been so much better. Patients should realise that any advice is given for their benefit.

A lady who once was a severely affected

osteoarthritis patient now comes to see me perhaps once every six months, just so that I can keep an eye on her. Unfortunately, she had lost two sisters who had died of heart failure after suffering from osteoarthritis. They were clear cases of poor oxygen transportation in the body, similar to the cause of death of Pope Paul.

Initially, her condition also deteriorated after beginning treatment. I clearly remember her husband coming to see me one Saturday morning requesting that he be told what in the world could be done for his wife. Would I please go over and talk to her. I went over later in the day to encourage her and, to convince her, I related a few case histories of patients who had been just like her. I told her that with constant effort and with a positive mind she would reach her goal.

I remember telling her a story I once heard in the United States. This story took place in the days of the gold rush and concerned an ambitious young man who had hit a very large strike. He formed a company and invested lots of money in machinery, convinced that the investment would pay off. They worked away at the mine until the rich vein suddenly disappeared totally. Everybody was called in to help relocate the vein, knowing that it definitely existed. However, there was no success. The expensive equipment, together with the mine, was sold and the new owner brought in a specialist to carry out a careful study. I seem to remember that I was told that the vein was found again approximately one foot from where the previous operation had stopped. The mine has since brought in millions of dollars. The first owner and founder of the mine had given up a little too soon.

I told this patient that if she ever considered giving up to think back to this story and to take heart from it; to always think that perhaps the next change of treatment might set her on the road to recovery. I don't know if the talk encouraged her, but it was obvious that she started to improve soon afterwards, so much so that she went with her husband to Australia for three months on holiday and returned renewed and happy. I sometimes remind her of this particular period in her life and how she has benefited from this experience in the long run.

I am often asked which methods of treatment I use. Not only do these vary from one patient to another, but frequently I also have to encourage these patients as best I can. As I have said before, we must look at every aspect of the case and treat every person as an individual. A few years ago I was asked to lecture on my approach to rheumatism and arthritis at a hospital for rheumatic diseases. There were quite a number of doctors present, among whom were some well-known rheumatologists.

After my talk there was deep silence and then the questions came.

The first question was: 'How in the world could I, through diet or through manipulative treatment, treat an arthritic hip?' I told them about the respected orthopaedic specialist who wrote to me asking if he might join me for a few days in my clinic. He was interested to see how I worked, for instance, with the hip joint, which was often still a mystery to him. I told him that it totally depended on the condition of the joint and of the patient. In some cases, as hip replacement operations are very successful, I might advise patients to take advantage of this opportunity. Before doing so, however, I will treat that hip with acupuncture and sometimes, if there is an inflammation, I will give mistletoe injections or, even better, enzyme injections. Immediately I got the answer: 'Oh, yes, the patient will be happy because when you give him acupuncture you release endorphins and encephalins – natural morphines – so, temporarily, patients will be happy. With your injections, you might temporarily relieve the pain too.'

With a real sense of achievement, though, I was able to tell him that I had many case histories on file of patients who had totally recovered with the help of a well-balanced diet and some homoeopathic remedies or perhaps some other therapy.

I told him about one particular gentleman who had first been in the care of an orthopaedic specialist and then went privately to a rheumatologist. Not having made any progress, he asked this specialist of he had his permission to see me, because he felt that he was too young for an operation. The rheumatologist agreed and I was later delighted when this particular specialist asked me what my treatment had been to warrant such improvement. I told him that this patient was following a specialised diet for arthritis and was given acupuncture treatment and enzyme injections.

The particular enzyme therapy I used for this patient consisted of Rheumajecta injections. I will try to explain the enzyme therapy in general and highlight Rheumajecta in particular.

Enzymes are active proteins which bring about all the reactions upon which life depends. Enzymatic activities take place according to biological needs. Enzymes control the metabolism of the endocrine and neuro-hormones. Since the neuro-hormonal system controls the production of enzymes in the whole of the organism, dysfunction can lead to multiple and diverse diseases.

Although not directly lethal, these pathological conditions rule out the harmonious development of the individual, either physically or psychically, and they provide the foundation for subsequent constitutional maladies which may lead to an earlier death.

Certain enzymes are capable of producing energy. Inadequate synthesis or disordered activity may lead to dysfunction of all organs and cause many complaints. It may be the cause of the disturbances. It should also be remembered that the whole metabolism of the cell is closely connected and therefore any functional disorder in one group of enzymes becomes cumulative throughout.

There are three consequences of enzymatic dysfunction, depending on the nature of the disturbance:

> deficiency or absence of metabolites;
> excess or accumulation of metabolites;
> abnormal metabolites,

All three are causal factors in a variety of complaints.

The fundamental principle of enzyme therapy is to treat the primary malfunction of a number of diseases for which, until recently, only symptomatic treatment was possible. This makes enzyme therapy a valuable new concept in modern medicine.

The pharmacodynamics of many drugs, including all tranquillisers and anti-histamine drugs, is based on the inhibition of enzymatic functions. It will, therefore, be readily understood that the supply of enzymes, together with their natural activators and inhibitors, into an organism deficient in them would be the therapy for many complaints. Enzyme therapy enables the organisms to combat illnesses with its own weapons by physiological means. Enzymology is a very complex science and the brief summary here is only an indication of the many complaints which can result from a deficient or imbalanced enzymatic activity.

We have looked at enzyme therapy in general. Now I will single out Rheumajecta from the various enzyme injection courses available, as this is the only relevant one in this context.

The only substances that muscles, nerves and joints have in common are mucopolysaccharides, the principal constituents of connective tissue and of periosteum. The periosteum is a fine film or membrane which completely covers each bone of the body.

Connective tissue is made up of a matrix of chondroitin sulphate sparsely beset with cells. Its function is to lend elastic support to blood vessels and nerves and to detoxicate serum permeating through the connective tissue. This tissue accompanies blood vessels and nerves right down to the smallest branches in the muscles and other organs.

Rheumajecta injections, which have no contra-indications or side effects, can be used for acute, sub-acute and chronic rheumatic infections of the muscles and joints. Even when patients have been on cortico-steroids this therapy proves very effective. After the first few treatments a definite improvement can be seen. This particular therapy has been a blessing for many patients.

My lecture on rheumatism and arthritis possibly created mixed feelings. Nevertheless there was a mutual understanding of the problems. Everyone felt that whether orthodox or alternative treatment was called for, all the rheumatic or arthritic patients deserved any help that was available.

Another question was raised. Did I believe that atmospheric conditions have an influence on the aches and pains of these patients? I told them about my old friend, Alfred Vogel, who was then well into his eighties. During his first visit to my clinic here in Scotland, he inquired as to how I was going to treat rheumatic or arthritic patients in this damp atmosphere. He gave me many suggestions and helpful advice on how to ease patients' conditions living in such a damp climate. I do believe that the cold and dampness does indeed have some bearing on the conditions of arthritic and rheumatic patients, but when we are aware of these influences something may be done to minimise the effects.

I told them about a severely crippled patient who

put the total blame for her condition on our climate. After gold and cortisone injections she eventually came to me for help. I was happy that I could quote to this gathering of doctors a few sentences from a letter she wrote me later, which read: 'I do not wish to wait till my next appointment to let you know that my pains have subsided. For the first time I spent a whole evening in a chair and felt comfortable about it. You know my condition only too well and therefore will realise what this means. I am grateful and indebted to you and look forward to my next treatment.'

This particular lady was in her eighties and in poor physical condition and yet she delighted me by being so happy and cheerful. She would tell me stories about the 'old people' in the Old Folk's Society, who were in fact all younger than she was.

Another 80-year-old osteoarthritic lady had gone through many different treatments before she came to see me. In a letter to me, she wrote: 'This has been my finest Christmas – I was able to do my own shopping for the first time in 28 years. My daughters join me in thanking you for all you have done for me.'

It is encouraging to see that older people, who could not be blamed if they gave up the struggle, have the courage to come and ask for help. Mostly they feel much better for it and are so grateful.

It is a treat to see some of the results which may be obtained with the help of various homoeopathic remedies. I remember a frail lady whose husband was a specialist in one of the big hospitals. She came to see me with a badly affected osteoarthritic neck and upper spine and was beyond acupuncture treatment due to extreme sensitivity. After we had a long talk I prescribed some homoeopathic powders for her. Later, her husband wrote to me to let me know how much his wife had benefited from this remedy and that she was free from pain for the first time for a long while. He suggested that as she was now so much better, she should return for some more treatment. We again see how the vital force in homoeopathic remedies can totally reverse a situation.

Osteoarthritis patients should be careful to avoid any wrenching and all exercises should be done gently. Sitting in the correct position is essential while gentle relaxation exercises are done, especially in the case of a stiff neck. Good footwear with leather soles should be worn by arthritic people, as we know that they often have a tendency towards flat feet or to cuboid problems. The type of floor in their home or their place of work is another important aspect, as it should conduct the flow of energy.

When I worked with Alfred Vogel in Switzerland

many years ago, we had an Italian lady working for us. She was a very hard worker, but unfortunately crippled with arthritis. I remember that Alfred Vogel did everything possible to help this lady but to little effect and she only just managed to keep going.

One day, when I went to collect something from the cellars, I saw her there. She was working in the department where the famous Herbamare salt is prepared. I asked her how frequently she worked in that department and she told me that she was there every day. I realised then why she did not improve – because this department had a cold concrete floor which totally cut off the energy flow. After she was moved to another department, we saw a miraculous improvement in her condition and she told me later, with great enthusiasm, how much better she felt ever since the change of job.

Sometimes it is necessary for osteoarthritic patients to follow a weight-reducing diet, but care should always be taken that anaemia does not result. I have seen some good long-lasting results where patients started off with a short fasting and cleansing diet. In such a diet it is advisable to have an enema during the first evening, before retiring to bed. Either warm water at body temperature may be used or a coffee enema. For two days, only have fresh fruit juices (not citrus fruit), herbal tea or vegetable juices for breakfast, lunch, dinner and supper. This particular fasting and cleansing diet may be followed up with the diet for rheumatoid arthritis explained in Chapter 1.

Let us look at the word 'arthritis'. This is a combination of two Greek words: *arthron* indicating joint and *itis* meaning inflammation.

With all inflammatory diseases careful preparations should take place before treatment begins, in order to gain the best outcome possible. Basic preparatory measures include cleansing and fasting in order to obtain proper bowel movements and a correct diet is important to aid detoxification. The body's immune system will be also be strengthened by these methods.

The success of treating osteoarthritic patients depends largely upon the degree of damage already done to the cartilage of the joints in question. However, if treatment is commenced in the early stages, success is much more likely if dietary advice is taken into consideration. Should manipulative treatment be necessary, the joint should be put through a range of gentle movements without causing any pain, so that the overall balance of the body and the spine is involved in the treatment. Frequently, when the whole spine is treated and in particular the upper part in the region of the ribcage, some restrictions may be eased. Careful cranial osteopathy can improve the flow of the cerebral spinal fluid. This, with some breathing exercises and lymph drainage, can help to ease pain and pressure in the joints and proves the benefits of oxygen.

We ought to take a lesson from the Chinese and Arabs in whose countries arthritis is unknown. They have stronger fingernails and healthy hair, because their food contains a good balance of silica, calcium and phosphorus. I have stated many times, in some of my earlier books, that this crippling disease is often caused by a poor diet and/or incorrect medicine.

A little bruise, swelling or a simple fracture are all indications that the affected bone or joint may become arthritic. In naturopathy we see, however, that if natural treatment is used, these may be brought under control quickly. Nature provides us with a whole range of suitable treatments which could be regarded as dietary supplements, such as celery, juniper, kelp or seaweed. All these rich sources of potassium or silica are freely available in nature. Considering this we can understand Jethro Kloss, who said:

> There is a science in nature,
> In trees, herbs, roots and flowers,
> Which man has not yet fathomed.

It is interesting to see how much nature has to offer in its natural products if, for example, we look at the effect of the Shark Liver Oil. My friend, Dr S.J.L. Mount, whom I regard as a great homoeopathic practitioner, did a marvellous trial on this and, since that time, for some rheumatoid arthritic patients, has had great results with this. The clinical trial report on Cho Jukai gives us the evidence.

Cho Jukai was the product name given to a shark liver oil preparation from Japan.

Cho Jukai is 99.7 per cent squalene, a liver oil obtained from deep water sharks, i.e. sharks that live beneath the sunlit layer of the sea. At this level, there is a distinct lack of oxygen, crushing water pressure and extreme cold. There is virtually no plant life or plankton, and creatures must adapt in order to survive. A feature of sharks existing under these conditions is that the liver, the most important organ of metabolism, accounts for about 25 per cent of body weight. Shark liver contains a great deal of oil, mostly squalene, which as unsaturated hydrocarbon combines to supply the tissues with oxygen. It is believed that squalene plays an important part in enabling the shark to range freely up and down the oceans and to survive at levels where there is little oxygen or food and under intense pressure, whereas other species are confined to one particular zone where pressure, light and temperature are more or less constant.

The action of squalene on ingestion by humans, if maintained, is to assist in supplying oxygen to the tissues of the body, expanding the blood vessels, improving circulation and respiration, and acting as a general tonic in relieving tiredness and stress. Squalene is also recommended as a safe, effective treatment for inflammatory conditions of the musculo-skeletal systems and gastro-intestinal tract.

For these reasons, Cho Jukai became a well-established health food supplement in Japan and its properties were increasingly studied and recognised by members of the medical and scientific professions in Japan.

Studies at the National Cancer Research Institute of Japan and at Hokushin General Hospital also suggested that squalene has anti-cancer activity and may provide immunity against some cancers. These findings were presented at the 4th International Symposium on the Prevention and Detection of Cancer (1980) held in London, and at the 4th World Congress of Cryosurgery, held in San Remo and published in the Japanese press in October 1980.

The study was carried out as a pilot study on the effects of shark liver oil on rheumatoid arthritis and one osteoarthritis case.

Method

Publicity was given to the trial and volunteers with rheumatoid arthritis were asked to apply to the London Natural Health Clinic.

Ten patients applied and were seen and examined to ensure the diagnosis. It turned out that the ten cases included nine with rheumatoid arthritis and one case with osteoarthritis. It was decided to run the trial as a straight study on these ten cases, each taking Cho Jukai (six capsules a day) over a two- to three-month period. The numbers were insufficient to plan a double blind trial.

The patients were given a full examination and blood tests were carried out to ascertain ESR and SCAT, and full blood count. They were then assessed as to the amount of pain they each had. This was carried out by means of the Ritchie Index. Using this Index, the affected joints were palpated by the examiner and the amount of reaction rated as follows:

0 – no pain experienced
1 – pain experienced
2 – pain experienced and patient winces
3 – pain experienced and patient withdraws affected limb.

This may sound crude as a scientific measurement but pain is notoriously difficult to measure and the

Ritchie Index if carried out by the same examiner gives good consistency and is used in arthritis trials throughout the world.

At the same time the patients were asked to fill in a form each day stating how much pain they had, how much inconvenience and stiffness and also how many painkillers they had taken. They were asked not to change their medication in any way but if they needed fewer painkillers as the trial went on, to note this on their form. They were then asked to give a final figure on the percentage improvement they thought they had achieved over the two- to four-month period and this corresponded usually very closely to the figure arrived at by the Ritchie Index. There was thus a subjective record and an objective one.

Results

Table 1 sets out the results of the trial with the comments of each patient recorded. An overall improvement figure is given which is the difference between the Ritchie Index at the first interview compared to the figure at the final interview.

This, however, is given for only those who completed the trial, as three of the ten dropped out. The average improvement in the pain experienced in the group of seven over the course of the trial was 59 per cent. This is seen in Table 2. This was a remarkably good figure and was certainly more than was expected when launching the trial. It would naturally be more satisfactory to run a double blind study and perhaps this will be possible as the next step. Interesting were the comments made by the patients as to the improvements in their general well being. Cho Jukai is supposed to improve the oxygenation and performance of most tissue cells and increase stamina and well being. The three patients who dropped out of the trial left for various reasons. One claimed he was allergic to the capsules. One had too much stress at home and had a flare-up of the arthritis probably as a consequence, and the third gave up after three weeks on the capsules as there was no improvement. Three weeks is really too short a time to assess effect.

TABLE 1

Seven cases that carried out trial treatment over a period of two to three months

A.B. Female, age 42, rheumatoid arthritis for 23 years. ESR 10, SCAT 1/400, later +VE. Wrists, hands, knees, toes affected. On Prednisolone 5 mg for eight months, wrists very swollen and methcarpal joints swollen and stiff. Ritchie Index initially 21.

1st Month

Reasonable improvement. Ritchie Index 11. Was doing well and then had a setback over Christmas following stress. A week without capsules and noticed the difference.

2nd Month

OK everywhere except left knee, wrists very good. An improvement all round. Ritchie Index 4.

3rd Month

Attempted to come off steroids and pain increased so resumed steroids. But overall improvement maintained. Ritchie Index 12.

Overall improvement in pain: 40 per cent.

J.D. Female, age 51. Rheumatoid arthritis for three years. ESR 16, later +VE. Shoulders, ankles, feet and hands affected. Takes Brufen and Acluagesic. Ritchie Index initially 19.5.

1st Month

More good days reported. Ritchie Index 19.5.

2nd Month

Ritchie Index 9.5.

3rd Month
Ritchie Index 3.5. Aches much better in morning. Dances every Saturday and very much better.

4th Month
Ritchie Index 1.5. Very good. Notices she can wear her shoes when dancing, much more easily. *Overall improvement in pain: 80 per cent.*

J.O. Male, age 42. Rheumatoid arthritis for ten years. ESR 12, SCAT 1/160. Both wrists and hands affected, ankles, neck, right knee which is worst affected. Joints swollen and deformed. Ritchie Index 9.

1st Month
Ritchie Index 2. Improving nicely.

2nd Month
Ritchie Index 6. Did have one or two attacks but longer periods of relief. A lot of difference overall. Can now manage gear levers with his hand and wrist. Neck better.

3rd Month
Ritchie Index 6. No more trouble in wrists. Left knee playing up a bit. Right knee bit swollen.

4th Month

Ritchie Index 0. Never felt so well. No problems with wrist. Has been altering his diet a little by cutting out coffee and white bread. Very pleased all round. *Overall improvement in pain: 100 per cent.*

A.B. Male, age 42. Rheumatoid arthritis for seven years. ESRG starting in fingers and knees, spreading to wrists, elbows ad shoulders. Hip and feet later affected. At the moment taking Indocid and gold. Gold stopped a month before trial. Ritchie Index 36.

1st Month

Ritchie Index 11.

2nd Month

Ritchie Index 1. Very much better. Feels stronger. Increased appetite. Getting through a night's work without painkillers. 'Terrific.' At times so well it defies description.

3rd Month

No further improvements but feels good. Doing things he hasn't done before. Nodules on hands and elbows disappearing. Can move joints more freely and close hand.

No painkillers at all. Ritchie Index 2.

4th Month
Improvement maintains.
Overall improvement in pain: 90 per cent.

W.S. Female, age 62. Rheumatoid arthritis for 24 years. ESR 21, SCAT 1/160. Condition began in feet, spread to wrists, ankles, shoulders, knees, fingers. Joints swollen and deformed. On 5 mg Prednisolone a day and painkillers. Ritchie Index 19.

1st Month
Ritchie Index 18.

2nd Month
Ritchie Index 13. Marked improvement. Even managing stairs better. 'Everybody has noticed.' In herself better and more relaxed. Appetite improving. Improved well being. Less painkillers.

3rd Month
Ritchie Index 12. Improvement maintained but experiencing a slight flare-up.
Overall improvement in pain: 37 per cent.

S.M. Male, age 43. Osteoarthritis for 15 years in cervical spine and shoulders. Stiffness and pain experienced in shoulder girdle. Ritchie Index initially 2.

1st Month
Ritchie Index 1. Remarkable changes. Has felt marvellous. Gives him a relaxation effect. Finds capsules a great help. Better than he has ever felt.

2nd Month
Ritchie Index 1. 'Capsules really wonderful.' More relaxed. A great change.
Overall improvement in pain: 50 per cent.

N.V. Female, age 20. Rheumatoid arthritis for 12 years. ESR 4. Arthritis started in wrists and ankles, spread to fingers, elbows and knees. Now also in hip and shoulder. Now on gold, Aloxpirin and physiotherapy. Ritchie Index initially 8.

1st Month
Ritchie Index 5. 'Up and down.' Fluctuating condition.

2nd Month
Ritchie Index 6. Feels capsules are doing her a little good. Shoulder slightly less stiff. Left knee still playing her up.
Overall improvement in pain: 25 per cent.

B.J. Female, age 51. Rheumatoid arthritis for 20 years. Did not come for second appointment as she stated she thought she was allergic to the capsules.

J.G. Male, age 48. Rheumatoid arthritis for 16 years. ESR 71, SCAT 1/64, later +VE. Did not come back for second appointment. Said he had tried capsules for three weeks with no improvement.

B.R. Female, age 48. Rheumatoid arthritis for 25 years. ESR 10. Swelling of feet, ankles, knees, fingers. Ritchie Index initially 17.

1st Month

Ritchie Index 13. First month was doing well and felt better. A setback was then suffered with a lot of psychological stress and patient felt unable to continue treatment.

Overall improvement in pain: 25 per cent.

TABLE 2

Case	Diagnosis	% improvement in pain	Time period
1. A.B.	R.A.	40	3 months
2. J.D.	R.A.	80	4 months
3. J.O.	R.A.	100	4 months
4. A.B.	R.A.	90	4 months

5. W.S.	R.A.	37	3 months
6. S.M.	O.A.	50	2 months
7. N.V.	R.A.	25	2 months

Overall average improvement: 59 per cent
Average time period: 3 months

Summary

Ten patients – nine with rheumatoid arthritis and one with osteoarthritis – were given Shark Liver Oil capsules (Cho Jukai) over a period of two to four months. Of the seven patients who completed the course a 59 per cent improvement in pain experienced was observed on the tests carried out.

3

Psoriatic Arthritis

THIS RHEUMATOID-LIKE arthritis, associated with psoriasis of the skin or nails, is a disease which we come across often, especially in the British Isles. Although psoriatic arthritis is often confused with psoriasis, there is a considerable difference between the two. For this reason I have decided to write about psoriasis in the last chapter of this book, and this chapter should be considered completely separate, as the two ought not to be confused.

As a rule, psoriatic arthritis is seen where the nails or skin are affected as a spin-off from arthritic joints. Inflammatory polyarthritis requires careful attention and with the help of X-rays it may be located exactly.

Although this disease seems akin to rheumatoid arthritis in many ways, it is less difficult to discover where the problems stem from and what kind of treatment is needed. Diet is particularly important in the treatment of psoriatic arthritis. For the first six to eight weeks, I usually advise that the following diet is adhered to, after which the diet for rheumatic arthritis (see Chapter 1) should be followed once the psoriasis-affected areas have cleared.

Diet for psoriatic arthritic people

Take only vegetables, especially raw. Dress salads with Molkosan (a milk-whey product). Use buttermilk, natural yoghurt (low fat), toasted wholemeal bread, cottage cheese, potatoes, Ryvita, sunflower or olive oil and honey.

Drink herbal teas, apple juice, blackcurrant juice, and natural brown rice, grapes and berries may all be eaten.

Do not use

Coffee, tea, white sugar or white flour (and products in which these are used); vinegar, tinned products, butter, cream, pork (sausages, bacon, ham, gammon, etc.), oranges, lemons, grapefruit, spices, mayonnaise, cucumber, tomatoes, cabbage, cauliflower, rhubarb or spinach. No sweets or chocolates and do not smoke or drink any alcohol.

General

Eat each day two plates of grated carrots and walk 1–1½ hours daily. One day per week should be a fasting day, when only apple juice, chamomile tea and carrot juice may be taken. Spend 15 minutes twice each day on deep breathing exercises before an open window or, if warm enough, outside.

Psoriatic arthritis is not easy to deal with, yet I have found over the years that if the patient co-operates there can be maximum benefits. The prescribed diets together with herbal medicine and acupuncture can result in excellent lasting improvement for the patient. With the psoriatic arthritic patient it is a matter of several body functions being out of balance. Once the balance is restored, the situation can be mastered and it is heartening to witness the results, even on severely affected patients.

Often, by the time I see these patients there is already long-standing damage. They might have suffered for years and have tried different cures, which have probably done them no good at all.

Immediate relief is sometimes obtained with the use of acupuncture. In the method of acupuncture taught by Dr Paul Nogier of Lyons, a dramatic body intelligence sends it messages to the right acupuncture points and acts as first aid before subsequent acupuncture treatments. This preliminary treatment will have a magnetic clinch on the tissues which have been constricting the offending joints and clogging up the circulation.

As a follow-up to the treatment of psoriatic arthritic patients, their emotional and physical ability should be studied and a way to balance body and mind should be sought. I have often witnessed a great self-pity, worry and sometimes bad temper in these patients, because of their unfortunate problem. It may take a little time before the patient is able to respond fully.

In the summer of 1975 a lady was carried into the surgery of my clinic in Preston. When I looked at her I thought of the possibility that she might die in my surgery. I had rarely seen such a severely crippled person and her joints were covered with an extremely unpleasant rash. She told me that it had all started with bouts of shivering and feeling ill. One morning, she collapsed in the kitchen. She was by then in constant pain and her skin was in a dreadful state. She decided to call her doctor, who prescribed her some drug treatment which gave her some relief, initially. She also bathed her skin as she had been advised. The lady was then referred to a consultant in one of the hospitals and underwent several tests. She was admitted to another hospital where more tests were done and X-rays were taken. She was informed that she had a blood disorder and that her spleen might have to be removed because of other complaints she suffered from besides psoriatic arthritis. However, she became so weak that an operation was not advised for the time being.

From her case history I learned that this lady had a very low count of white blood cells and that all her food had to be liquidised as her jaws would not open fully. There was nowhere left for her to turn and a friend had made an appointment for a consultation with me. She showed herself willing to follow my instructions, which were mainly about her dietary habits, and I suggested some herbal medicine.

It did not happen overnight, but she boasts that she is now capable of doing most things for herself again. Her problems have largely cleared up and she can manage to go up and down the stairs by herself. She also bathes herself again, which had been unthinkable for years. I still see her occasionally and it always delights me to see her mobile. Acupuncture, herbal medicine and dietary control – all combined – solved most of her problems.

A comprehensive vitamin, mineral and trace element regime should be followed by psoriatic arthritic patients. A good multi-vitamin is recommended, together with minerals such as calcium, magnesium and silicium. A selection of amino acids is also helpful and in certain circumstances biochemical salts such as Natrum Muriaticum 6x and Kalium Sulphur 6x.

I recall another psoriatic arthritic patient who came to me in a poor condition. I examined him before deciding upon the treatment to recommend and asked him what his occupation was. He told me that he was a taxi driver in one of the bigger cities. Immediately I thought of all the petrol fumes and exhaust gases which could be the cause of lead poisoning. Before I started him on any treatment. I gave him a homoeopathic lead antidote, which resulted in dramatic improvement. He then started on his dietary regime and received acupuncture treatment. I also suggested using Joint Mobility Factors and a herbal tea such as Golden Grass to cleanse the kidneys.

Finally, I recommended a high dosage of vitamin C. The patient absolutely thrived on this treatment.

When I see him from time to time, he tells me how he is very grateful that he was able to resume full work again. I am fully convinced that the turning point in this case was the homoeopathic remedy, which cleared his blood from the poisoning that had gradually taken place over the years.

This case reminds me of another patient, this time

from Wales. This particular gentleman was almost crippled and his joints were covered with a rash. I prescribed the same herbal regime for him and introduced him to Oil of Evening Primrose. I have written in detail about Oil of Evening Primrose in my book *New Developments in Multiple Sclerosis*, yet here I want to stress again the beneficial properties of this plant with its attractive little yellow flowers.

The extract of this wonderful plant not only eases the pains in the nerves, but strengthens both the brain and nerves. We also know that the Evening Primrose oil stimulates the liver, spleen and digestive system and therefore helps these arthritic conditions.

The Evening Primrose plant contains a good quantity of magnesium and iron and is also rich in selenium, which is often deficient in our soil. Wherever the primrose grows wild, selenium is present in the soil. We know that selenium, like vitamin E, is a powerful anti-oxidant and because the two are synergistic, they work better together. A deficiency of vitamin E or selenium may cause an accumulation of cholesterol in the muscles.

We also know that this plan has a special resonance with the human body and its blood. Its gamma-linoleic acid plays an important role in the treatment of psoriatic arthritis. A series of controlled studies in the Department of Dermatology at the

University of Bristol, using double-blind tests and involving both adults and children, demonstrated that Evening Primrose oil produced significant improvements without any side effects.

Even in the olden days significant results in the treatment of arthritis and related diseases were obtained with hydrotherapy or water treatments. The water treatment using Austrian mud, for example, has been used in clinics for many years. Recently, I have been doing trials with a water treatment using Dead Sea mineral salts. This healing method from the Dead Sea is ideally suited to rheumatism and arthritis patients. Psoriatic arthritic patients in particular have benefited substantially.

This is not a new treatment, as the Romans already knew about the extraordinary powers of the Dead Sea mineral salts 2,000 years ago. The Roman historian Josephus Flavius wrote: 'Travellers take home as much of the salt as they can, for it brings to the human body a cure, and is therefore used in many medicines.'

Much earlier still, the Jewish kings, David and Solomon, and the Queen of Sheba, a woman of legendary beauty, built curative bathing palaces on the shores of the Dead Sea. These were forerunners to the modern spas, where sufferers from skin problems, rheumatism and arthritis have found much relief.

The sea (really a vast inland lake) is unique in a number of ways. Lying 1,300 feet below sea level, it is the lowest place on earth and also one of the hottest. The intense heat of the sun causes continuous evaporation of the sea water, resulting in a massive 28 per cent concentration of mineral salts – seven times that of the world's oceans. Indeed, as is well known, the Dead Sea is so full of mineral salts and is so naturally buoyant that if you bathe in it you can't sink. It is amusing to float on the surface of the water reading a book or sipping a drink, but swimming is scarcely possible and not particularly enjoyable because of the intense saltiness. You don't bathe for pleasure but for other benefits.

The Dead Sea's remarkable properties, known for so many centuries but only recently confirmed by scientific studies, are due to a unique combination of 41 different minerals found in the salts. These derive from numerous springs which flow into the sea from the surrounding mountains. Nowhere else in the world do these natural minerals combine in a similar amalgam. A typical sample of Dead Sea mineral salts contains heavy concentrations of magnesium and potassium chloride with lesser amounts of calcium and sodium in the form of bromides, chlorides and sulphates. These natural concentrates are used world wide both for the treatment of arthritis and for sufferers from psoriasis, an unsightly skin condition that affects millions of people.

The International Psoriasis Centre was located at the Dead Sea. A great deal of scientific work has been done there to establish the effects of treatment with the mineral salts. One leading authority, Prof. Shani of the Hebrew University in Jerusalem, has said that in his view the components found in the salts represent 'the most important factor in the successful treatment of psoriasis and psoriatic arthritis'.

Other international scientists have published the results of clinical trials showing a high success rate. Intractable skin problems such as eczema, rashes and dry patches caused by exposure to the sun have all responded well to treatment, it has been reported in various medical papers.

Tests on patients suffering from arthritis and rheumatism have shown improvements ranging from increased strength of grip to improved mobility of limbs. Most patients have reported less pain in response to treatment at Dead Sea spas. This has led health authorities in some European countries to send selected patients for a month's treatment – all expenses paid. They find that this costs less than treating them in hospital back home.

No harmful effects have been reported during the many years of clinical trials. Indeed, as in all other forms of alternative medicine, one of the greatest advantages of the mineral salts is that there are none of the risks associated with the use of drugs.

A trip to the Dead Sea is beyond most of us, unfortunately. However, the minerals extracted from the sea for use at the spas are now available in a number of clinics in this country. They can also be obtained in small packs for self-treatment at home. This involves bathing either the whole body or just the affected parts in a small amount of the salts dissolved in warm water.

Dead Sea mud, which contains the same minerals, has similar soothing and healing properties. Many people use it to relieve aching joints. It has also proved helpful for treating difficult skin problems, particularly those on the scalp.

The response of patients to treatment in British clinics and at home ranges from slight but heartening improvement to quite remarkable relief from persistent problems. In my experience, the healing power of the Dead Sea is much more than just an ancient legend.

For those who wish to treat themselves with Dead Sea mineral salts at home, the instructions are as follows:

Psoriatic Arthritis

Day 1

1 Dissolve one bag of mineral salts in 5 litres (8 pints) of water at body temperature (37-38 C) placed in a foot bath or bowl.

2 Immerse inflamed joint (i.e. hand and wrist or foot and ankle) for 20 minutes.

3 Remove limb from water – SAVE WATER.

4 Carefully rinse limb to remove all mineral salts.

5 Dry carefully.

6 Wrap the treated limb in a warm towel or blanket and relax for half an hour, keeping the limb warm and at rest in a comfortable position.

Day 2

No treatment.

Day 3

1 Reheat the mineral-salt water saved from the first day to 3738 C.

2 Follow instructions 2 to 6 as for Day 1.

Day 4

No treatment.

Day 5

Exactly as Day 3. Now throw away the mineral-salt water.

Day 6

No treatment.

Day 7

No treatment.

Day 8

Start the whole week's regime again.

Repeat until four weeks' treatment has been completed.

This treatment is beneficial for psoriatic arthritis patients and totally safe as there are no side effects.

4

Polyarthritis

A CONSULTANT rheumatologist wrote in a letter to the general practitioner of one my patients: 'This lassie with sero positive polyarthralgia seems extraordinarily well with little stiffness. I am delighted that she has managed to maintain her current condition without long-term treatment. She only complains of a sore throat at present and I doubt that this is in any way related to her arthritis. I understand that she is under treatment and have arranged to review her condition in about twelve months' time. If her condition remains quiescent, we shall then discharge her.'

How happy I was that by a coincidence I chanced

to read this letter. I remember when I saw the girl
first and her state at that time. The various drugs
she had been prescribed had been to no avail, and
she had done everything within her power to
improve her condition. The letter stated rightly that
her sore throat was still present, but missed the fact
that this was actually the cause of her polyarthritic
condition. Knowing this helps us to realise that
polyarthritis should not be underestimated and that
there are various reasons why this condition can
develop. This particular girl displayed quite a
number of symptoms which could have been
attributed to polyarthritis.

What exactly is polyarthritis, a condition which is
indeed so often misunderstood? Unfortunately,
there are not many publications available which are
devoted to this disease. It is correctly classified as a
partially or completely arthritic disease. The
distressing aspect of polyarthritis is that it affects
nearly all the joints, which makes it very hard to
bear.

The incidence of polyarthritis is a lot worse, in my
opinion, in the Netherlands than here in Britain,
although here too I come across it often enough. It
is mainly the younger generation who are supposed
to be affected by polyarthritis and unfortunately I
must say that this confirms my own experience.

Younger polyarthritic patients seem to benefit

greatly from enzyme therapy. I remember a newly married young lady who was suffering from various ailments. Her consultant agreed with me that this looked very much like a case of polyarthritis. The acute pain made any movement of the joints very difficult. As a result, when she walked she seemed to be swaying from side to side, as one imagines a drunken sailor would. She followed the enzyme therapy and, rather than injections, I recommended pills which I obtained from Germany and she showed incredibly good results within two weeks. After that, I also gave her some Vogel remedies and her illness almost disappeared.

I had heard that she had given birth to a daughter and a few years later I chanced to meet her again. I immediately became aware from the way she was walking that her condition had worsened. I asked her if she was doing anything to improve her condition and she said that she had been considering coming to see me again following a recent deterioration in her condition.

When I questioned her I discovered that she was not paying any attention to her diet and that she had been mixing carbohydrates and proteins haphazardly. It did not take very long for her to improve after she took my advice to immediately correct her dietary habits. We know that polyarthritis is a problem to be reckoned with and to wilfully neglect or ignore dietary instructions seems always to aggravate matters.

There are many ways to approach polyarthritis, but before I go into more detail about possible treatment methods, I would like to look in general at this particular arthritic condition. It is often thought that a number of toxins or micro-organisms are responsible for this particular problem. I have frequently noticed increased toxicity in the blood of polyarthritic patients. There could also be a family history of some form or another, especially in cases of chronic polyarthritis. Where in the case of the previously mentioned patient, chronically suppurating tonsils were at the root of the illness, teeth, gums or roots have also been known to be the cause.

Not only can the joints be affected by polyarthritis, but the same may happen to the heart and sometimes the condition deteriorates very quickly indeed. Aspirin is generally prescribed, or other anti-inflammatory drugs, and we find that gastric troubles, head noises and dizziness often follow, due to an excess of aspirin. If the ailment worsens, the doctor or specialist will prescribe cortisone or ACTH. These remedies might give temporary relief, but many eventually cause the patient's condition to deteriorate and the problem will increase tenfold if osteoporosis sets in.

There are several suitable methods to treat this condition. Of course I would recommend the arthritis diet as detailed in Chapter 1. Certain remedies such as Symphosan, Petasites, Arnica Gel and St John's Wort Oil have been responsible for good improvements. Alfred Vogel writes in his book, *The Nature Doctor*, that mud cures, Turkish baths or mineral baths have also proven very helpful to these patients.

As with any person suffering from arthritis-related conditions, the polyarthritic patient needs to be looked at as a whole person and the system may be cleansed with the use of herbs. It is sometimes difficult to understand why people do not take a lesson from nature and use herbal medicine to ease these crippling and debilitating conditions. Herbs are safe and gentle and it is interesting to see how every herb has a specific role to perform in herbal medicine.

Should the polyarthritis have been caused by a chronic catarrhal condition or an infection of the tonsils, dietary measures will have to be employed to remove any toxicity from the bloodstream as these toxins might have been the cause of the original problem. In those instances homoeopathic remedies come in very useful.

Definite attention should be given to the source of the infection. Not only the teeth and tonsils, but even the appendix, could be a contributory factor and these areas should all be treated. Under these conditions acupuncture should not be overlooked, especially when there is a doubt about the blood supply. Any contraction or tension can distort the flow affecting every part of the body immediately a nerve stimulates muscular contractions. Once the alignment of bone structure is disturbed, it ceases to operate on the spring of an anti-magnetic basis. This force then becomes short-circuited and the magnetic force takes over, jamming the joints, stiffening the tissues and affecting the circulation. Pain spasms follow and the arthritis gets worse. When we correct the anti-magnetic forces, either by exercises or by acupuncture, the situation can be reversed. Gentle exercise is most important to ease the circulation flow and strengthen the tissues.

Polyarthritis patients have also found relief from the use of Oil of Evening Primrose, especially if combined with fish-oil supplements. It is claimed that if our eating habits resembled that of the Eskimo, there would be no complaints of rheumatism or arthritis, as it has been discovered that fish-oil supplements might reduce stiffness or pain in the joints. I suppose this is possibly the reason why in olden days cod liver oil was used so frequently. A product called Marlinol is now available, which combines these two oils in the correct proportions.

A study was done some years ago at the Albany Medical College in New York, involving an experiment to reduce the level of cholesterol in the blood. During the trials, neither doctors nor patients knew who was receiving active treatment with polyunsaturated fatty acids combined with a diet high in polyunsaturates, and who was not. After three months on this particular diet, patients had fewer tender joints and suffered less stiffness than others who were on a diet high in saturated fats. When they were taken off their polyunsaturated diet for a period of time, the number of tender joints started to increase again. These results underline the importance of combining diet and harmless natural and herbal remedies in the treatment of arthritic complaints.

We ought to learn to live according to the laws of nature and follow a good nutritional programme. The correct acid/alkaline balance will help the stiff and aching bodies almost right away. I have found also with polyarthritis patients that a vitamin therapy is most important, together with possibly some cod liver oil or individually prescribed homoeopathic or herbal remedies. Some general recommendations are to drink mineral water; use salt sparingly; delete sugar and ban citrus fruits from the diet.

The vitamin therapy which I often use is as follows:

Vitamin A	10,000 i.u.
Vitamin D	400 i.u.
Vitamin B complex	75 mg
Vitamin B3, Niacin	100 mg twice daily
Vitamin B5	500 mg
Vitamin C	
– (sustained release)	2 gr
Vitamin E	400 i.u.
Lecithin granules	2 tbsp daily
Bromelain	200 mg
Urticalcin	6 tablets
High balance chelated mineral formula	

A letter reached me from a Harley Street specialist regarding a mutual patient. This patient had consulted me and made his appointments to coincide with his frequent visits to Scotland. He was delighted with his improvement and felt generally much more supple. His specialist wrote: 'I, too, am most impressed with what you have accomplished in just a few visits. I am concerned, though, what action should now be taken. Would you please give me some guidance so that we may keep this patient in his present state of health.'

Such letters are obviously most encouraging, especially when they come from doctors or practitioners who have opened their minds to the fact that complementary medicine or, rather, naturopathy, offers us many alternative ways of treatment. With pleasure I realise that in recent years the gap is getting smaller, which is all to the benefit of the alleviation of human suffering.

5

Gout

GOUT IS AN intensely painful disease which often attacks small joints, especially those in the toes. The victims of this affliction are mostly male. We often see reference to gout in historical books. In the Bible we read that in his old age King Asa of Judah was crippled by a foot disease. This very possibly was gout.

Gout was supposed to have been more common among people who could afford rich foods. Today, many people can afford food which is too rich for their own good and they might suffer an attack of gout. When the uric acid levels are high, the blood cannot contain the solution. Uric acid will start its crystallisation process and the lymphocytes – the white blood cells whose job it is to remove the foreign matter – attack these crystals. The uric acid crystals will be enveloped by lymphocytes, which attempt to break them down chemically and digest them. This is totally impossible as the sharp crystals rupture the cells and destructive liquids are released, destroying the cell itself and also surrounding cells.

The fluids released from the white cells attack the bone joints causing the gouty arthritis and considerable swelling. Gout may be caused by an inherent defect of purine metabolism in which uric acid appears in excess in the tissues. The resulting attacks are extremely painful and occur most often in the joints of the big toe.

However, not all hyperuricaemic people develop gout. It depends totally on the circumstances. With acute gout, we witness its appearance without any forewarning. Occasionally it may be caused by slight trauma like ill-fitting shoes, over-indulgence in alcohol, emotional stress or infection; or, even worse, it may be due to over-use of penicillin, insulin or mercurial diuretics. The onset may appear after excess of any of these particular elements. We know that the causes of gout have not changed drastically over the centuries and that a diet where the acid/alkaline level is disturbed is frequently the cause of acute inflammatory response.

We notice only too often the first symptoms of gout in the osteopathic department of our clinic. These symptoms may be discovered by looking at the skin of the big toe, which can be tense, hot or shiny. Acute attacks of gout usually last a few days and may or may not persist in gouty arthritis. They are, however, a definite warning that diet should be looked at. We do find that people who are particularly prone to these attacks tend to eat a lot of purine-rich foods, such as meat, fish, chocolate, peanuts, alcohol and often too much sugar and salt. Smoking, which is also a contributory factor, comes under this category too. Usually, when these symptoms and warning signals are present we try to adjust the patient's diet. If we get the necessary co-operation it is wonderful to see how gratefully the body reacts. The symptoms sometimes disappear very quickly after minor dietary adjustments have taken place.

In cases of chronic gout, however, things are a little bit more difficult. Attacks occur not only in the usual places, but the small joints in the hands and feet may also be affected and sometimes the shoulders, the cervical spine and even the sacro-iliac joint.

With chronic gout drastic action should be taken. I remember a businessman who was plagued by this problem (which should not be confused with either rheumatoid or osteoarthritis) and asked me for advice. He was really suffering and, not knowing what to do, compounded his miseries by eating all the wrong things. Moreover, he drank more alcohol than he was accustomed to in order to try and forget his sorrows, which he thought were caused by rheumatoid arthritis.

However, he definitely suffered from gouty arthritis. I advised him to stop taking any alcohol or tobacco and to remove from his diet all the foods which were making his condition worse. I also gave him some remedies including Knotgrass Complex, Solidago Complex and Joint Mobility Factors. Thankfully, after a short time, his trouble decreased and when I last heard from him he told me how well he was and how grateful for all the good advice on his now sensible lifestyle.

In cases of gout, I mostly advise an increased fluid intake, especially with patients who have a tendency to form stones as a result of uric acid. These patients should take great care that their kidneys are not damaged. They should drink lots of fluid and once a week have a fasting day. As already mentioned, a fasting diet with plenty of liquid to drink will be helpful and relive the pain quickly.

Although it sounds incredible, it is claimed that almost 10 per cent of mankind are afflicted with this painful disease. I personally think that this percentage is an exaggeration as gouty arthritis is often confused with other kinds of arthritis, and vice versa, but we do know that more people suffer from this disease than we can possibly imagine.

The only way to treat this dreadful affliction is by adjusting the diet. Diets which are suitable for this problem have already been mentioned in previous chapters.

As I have already suggested for arthritis, a very good remedy indeed is to drink, every morning, the juice of a raw potato. Some people find this extremely difficult to swallow, but it is so beneficial and a treatment that everyone can afford. Prepare and drink it fresh first thing in the morning. I advise patients with gout, too, to take a handful of mustard seeds with it and they will soon notice a change for the better.

An after-effect of gouty arthritis is that the patient has a tendency to develop a degree of arteriosclerosis. Although arteriosclerosis in layman's terms is called the hardening of the arteries, we also have learned that it is extremely important for the arteriosclerotic patients to remove high cholesterol foods from their diets to eliminate the production of uric acid. It is not the jelly-like cholesterol which deposits itself on the inside walls of the artery which does the most serious damage. The particles within the artery itself pose a much greater problem and these are often caused by smoking and drinking. When they are calcified, all sorts of problems can occur and the result could even be a brain haemorrhage.

If this tendency exists with patients, it is very important to prescribe chelation therapy, which may be applied by injections. Nowadays an oral chelation is also available. This therapy, whether oral or intravenous, contains vitamins, minerals, trace elements and other valuable ingredients which try and dissolve not only the cholesterol, but also the more serious, calcified particles within the arteries.

I cannot stress sufficiently the importance of the difference between the major groups of arthritis and I would very much emphasise that the investigations which are done should be totally in accordance with the symptoms and background problems, as X-ray plates do not always give us the right picture.

In homoeopathic and herbal medicine some wonderful remedies exist to help the gouty arthritis patient. To my thinking the most important of them all is comfrey (*Symphytum officinalis*). This remedy has been used since ancient times and in the treatment of gout today it can be used in several forms. I prefer to use the remedy Symphosan, which is a combination of:

Symphytum officinalis	Comfrey
Hamamelis virginiana	Witch hazel
Hypericum perforatum	St John's Wort
Solidago virginiana	E. Golden Rod
Saninclua europea	E. Sanicle
Sempervivum tectorum	Houseleek
Arnica montana	Arnica

This remedy, only available from a practitioner, is absolutely marvellous for arthritic distortions and swollen joints.

Great results may be obtained if the painful area, which usually is the big toe, is treated locally with comfrey. Take a raw root, grate it finely and apply to the affected area in the form of a poultice. If it is impossible to obtain a root, then a tincture of comfrey may be spread lightly on the affected parts. Do take care, however, not to massage in this tincture, but just gently dab it on, as this is most beneficial. This treatment may be followed by clay or cabbage poultices and is a marvellous help in cases of gouty arthritis.

An extremely effective way to suppress the uric acid level is by using A.Vogel Solidago Complex which can be used safely to rid the body of excess fluid. *Solidago virgaurea* (Golden Rod) has important anti-inflammatory, antispasmodic and antiseptic action. It soothes irritations in the urinary tract caused by infections such as cystitis and uerthritis, and both prevents the formation and facilitates the elimination of kidney stones.

Solidago vigaurea, Betula pendula (Birch), *Ononis spinosa* (Restharrow) and *Equisetum arvense* (Horsetail), all of which are in Solidago Complex, contain saponins, flavonoids and tannins. Their diuretic action is the result of the saponins and flavonoids. Saponins are also anti-inflammatory and tannins are astringent.

To refer back to the dietary considerations – we should be very careful with acid-forming foods, e.g. meat, especially sausages, processed meats, bacon and ham, processed food in general; animal fat; white flour, sugar (particularly white sugar); citrus fruit, such as oranges, grapefruit, lemons, tangerines and clemetines; tomatoes, potatoes aubergines and peppers. Onion or garlic, however, are excellent to reduce the extreme pain gout patients suffer occasionally. Once more I must warn these patients against a protein-rich diet. Not only the foods which I have already mentioned are unsuitable for them, but also dairy products like eggs, cheese, milk and milk products. They should also be wary of including peas, beans and lentils in their diet.

I can safely say that if the gouty arthritis patient adheres to the advice given in this chapter, within two to three months the symptoms will disappear. In my honest opinion, the foods mentioned above should be crossed off their diet for the rest of their lives.

Natural remedies combined with the recommended diet will be followed by a healing process and there is nothing so gratifying as the body repaying you with good health. This can be achieved if dietary corrective measures are taken and adhered to and the result will be a better quality of life.

6

Ankylosing Spondylitis or Marie Struempell Disease

A YOUNG MAN told me some time ago: 'I don't have what you would call a serious problem and I suppose I could learn to live with it, if it does not get any worse.' Seemingly his condition had started to deteriorate recently and that was the reason he came to see me, as his wife had told him that it might be just a case of vitamin deficiency or something similar. When I examined the young man I realised that it was nothing as simple as that and that we had quite a problem on our hands. The gentleman concerned suffered from a disease called Ankylosing Spondylitis.

We know this to be a chronic progressive disease of the small joints in the spine. It always amazes me that this particular condition finds its victims mostly in young men and how quickly it can spread from one joint of the spinal column to another. A lesion may occasionally be the cause of this disease, in which case it may be contained, but generally it tends to be a progressive disease.

The young man did not seem unduly worried about his condition and I told him which ways were open to us to arrest this process. Here I could draw on previous experience. I have treated many people, young and old alike, whose spines were completely bent and who suffered typical rheumatoid arthritis symptoms.

This condition may result from an infection which could be inactive for a long time before pain and stiffness starts, mostly in the lower back area. It progresses up the spine, affects the region of the chest and neck and may progress to the shoulders. The bones of the spine stiffen and there is a danger that total mobility may disappear. The patient's head gradually begins to poke forward. The upper spine stiffens and also bends forward, so that the poor person is always looking at the ground as he or she is unable to straighten up fully.

Ankylosing Spondylitis sometimes brings immense psychological problems as people gradually lose their mobility and become invalids. However, because this disease usually strikes the younger generation, more specifically young men between 20 and 40, they often have the will to get better and turn out to be marvellous patients to work with.

Another young man came to see me with a severely affected spine. The disease was in a very progressive state, yet he had an iron will and he placed himself in my hands, giving me his total co-operation. However, he was very afraid of needles and although I assured him that there would be no pain, he preferred not to have any acupuncture treatment. I told him that we would start his treatment with a healthy diet, as mentioned in Chapter 1. I then prescribed a nosode therapy to try and remove the original infection and gradually introduced some herbal homoeopathic remedies. I also advised him to undertake some hydrotherapy treatment.

Over the years the disease in this young man has never progressed any further. In fact, he has steadily improved. He and his wife have had two children in the meantime, which goes to show that he is now capable of leading a normal life. Once in a while he comes to see me again. This usually happens when he has been overdoing things or has done some heavy lifting and as a result his spine is painful again.

On one of these occasions he asked me for some acupuncture treatment as he was sure that it would ease the pain. This shows not only his increased confidence, but also that when in pain a patient will sacrifice almost any fear in order to get help. He now knows from experience that acupuncture does not hurt and that it is definitely beneficial to him. Suffice to say, he now has acupuncture treatment whenever it is considered necessary.

I remember that he came to show me their second baby shortly after it was born and happily acknowledged that if he had not persevered he would be like some of his fellow-sufferers, who were completely helpless. This goes to show that even with a serious condition such as Ankylosing Spondylitis one should never give up, because if we work at it there is always hope.

Calcification is a particular problem with this disease and at a later stage it may develop into ossification. It is because of this danger that I am not in favour of any osteopathic treatment for Ankylosing Spondylitis patients.

A far better way to treat this disease is with a sensible diet, as recommended for the rheumatoid arthritis patients. Internal and external use of Comfrey Cream is very helpful, as well as Knotgrass Complex and the green-lipped mussel extract.

Immediately after diagnosis a programme of

gentle exercises should be embarked upon, to help the patient to try to remain as supple as possible and maintain movement in the joints. Relaxation is of the utmost importance to try and relieve muscle spasms. It is essential that the patient is in a comfortable position before commencing relaxation exercises.

One simple but effective exercise can be done as follows: while standing straight with the back against a wall, go down gently, letting the knees bend and trying to keep the back against the wall. Slowly straighten up again, with the help of a chair in front if needed. Exercises are of great help in arresting this condition. It is also advisable for these patients to lie or sleep supine on a good firm mattress.

Breathing exercises are also necessary. As the disease progresses, the joints of the thorax or chest tend to calcify and limit the amount of air which can enter the lungs. Deep breathing should be encouraged, using as much chest expansion as possible. However, once the chest has become rigid the Hara breathing exercises (explained in my book, *Stress and Nervous Disorders*) are of great assistance to keep the lungs ventilated. They are best done on the floor.

In some cases, hydrotherapy treatments such as hot baths or hot packs of kaoline poultices on the very sore parts will prove helpful. Sometimes when I look at these bent and stiffened spines, I am reminded of how, as a young boy, I would sit for hours with little frogs and play with them. I used to hold them in the palm of my hand and with a little push of their feet they would straighten their legs and jump away, using the same movement as they would when leaping along the ground – with very little muscular contraction.

In acupuncture it is interesting to see how the electrical energy force, or 'spring' in the joints, can be generated into the acupuncture points where it relaxes the contraction and also how these little needles, through the brain, do their work. The stiffened joints can start to work again thanks to this extra energy force. As with those little frogs – where the timing of their action was all important – the same principle of accuracy applies to acupuncture.

A widespread misunderstanding persists that does can move. It is, however, the muscle which moves the bone and one thing leads to another. If we throw a pebble into a pool of water, the circles in the water are noticeable long after the pebble has sunk. In the same way, acupuncture treatment will have lasting effects for the Ankylosing Spondylitis patient. Because the alignment of the bone structure has been disturbed and the 'spring' has gone from the joints, some extra energy force is needed to loosen these stiffened joints and stimulate the circulation in the tissue.

Endorphins and encephalins are released during acupuncture treatment and these will act to ease the pain. We often find that the pain in these stiffened joints can be eased with the aid of acupuncture or biomagnetic therapy.

Biomagnetic therapy is becoming more and more popular as a way of correcting the antimagnetic forces which sometimes operate in the joints and it is beneficial to all arthritic patients. To the stiffened, sometimes even useless joints of the Ankylosing Spondylitis patient the results are often amazing. There are cases when it seems almost impossible to get any movement in these almost hardened and totally stiffened joints; it is here that the energy vibration therapy really comes into its own.

For these patients we may use the biomagnetic or magneto-magnetic therapy. In the magneto-magnetic fields of living systems (including human beings), two poles provide totally different effects when applied to living biological matter such as cell tissue and/or organs. We all know that blood cells, where the selective membrane separates the biological changes, provide positive and negative action or, as it is often termed, an action of potassium positive and sodium negative ions. It is also known that these two potential force fields present themselves completely differently when magneto-magnetic energies are applied.

I have often proved that when these magnets are used correctly, i.e. with the north and south pole in the right positions, the resulting magnetic energies will facilitate correction of the anti-magnetic forces. Although there is a degree of misunderstanding on this particular point, it is true to say that the north pole of a magnet will always seek the south pole. This has resulted in the development of the theory that the south pole offers a positive form of energy and that the north pole provides a negative form of energy. We look for the south-pole end of the magnet and obtain the right spin of electrons.

When working with copper and zinc magnets it is interesting to see that positive always looks for negative and that by using these with body energy on certain acupuncture points, the results are sometimes amazing. The British Biomagnetic Association is doing marvellous work in this field and, using these low-cost magnets, especially copper and zinc magnets, it has often justifiably been said that 'all life is energy and all energy is vibration'.

Whenever I see people with this dreadful disease, who have been my patients for years and have been able to keep going with increased mobility, I am always reminded of a cheerful young Ankylosing Spondylitis patient, whom I saw every couple of months. He never failed to tell me how wonderful it was to be without pain and to be able to do a full day's work and care for his family. He considered it a small sacrifice to have to follow a reasonably strict diet. He also used Symphosan and from time to time had acupuncture treatment. I also gave him an occasional magnetomagnetic therapy treatment, which gave him back that little bit of 'spring' which he had missed for a number of years.

This disease and others which often affect people before the age of 40, in the prime of their life, make me feel grateful that we have learned ways to help those who suffer. I have said that in magneto-magnetic therapy, positive always looks for negative and the same is relevant in the emotional field. A positive attitude can overcome negative thoughts and bring back some happiness, which makes the quality of life so much better.

7

Still's Disease –
Juvenile Rheumatoid Arthritis

Paget's Disease –
Osteitis Deformans

STILL'S DISEASE and Paget's disease would have
very little in common if it were not for the fact that
the incidence of both has risen in recent years. As
the one disease affects young children and the other
disorder older people, I feel that both deserve a little
attention in this book.

Still's disease is a juvenile rheumatoid arthritis. It
occurs mainly in children and resembles the adult
version. This disease affects the larger joints and

interferes with the growing and development process of the child. There are several ways in which this disease manifests itself.

Although the disease has unpleasant symptoms for the child, the prognosis is more favourable for a youngster than for an adult. In most cases a remission will take place.

However, during all my years of practice I have seen many children affected by this particular disease and have been worried and sometimes very sad to watch the development. It breaks my heart to see young children in my surgery who are diagnosed to be suffering from this Still's disease. Unfortunately, I have seen over the past years that aspirin, however well tolerated, as well as cortisone, has often caused lasting growth problems in children. This goes to show how careful we have to be with the use of drugs. For children who tend to be scared of most forms of treatment, a choice to suit the individual can be made from the different methods available.

Iris diagnosis, which is a marvellous way of diagnosing through the eyes, provides us with the finely tuned analyses of the patient's biochemistry and of emotional and circumstantial factors which are hard to determine by any other method. Iridology is the science of analysing the delicate structures of the iris in the eye. Under the magnification of biomicroscope, the iris reveals itself as a world of minute details, or a complete map that represents a communications system capable of handling an astonishing quantity of information.

The iris is an extension of the brain, prolifically endowed with hundreds of thousands of nerve endings, microscopic blood vessels, muscle and other tissue. Each iris is connected to every organ and tissue of the body by way of the brain and nervous system. The nerve fibres receive their impulses by way of the optic nerve, optic thalamus and spinal cord and are formed embryologically from mesoderm and neuroectoderm tissues. Both the sympathetic and parasympathetic nervous systems are present in the iris. In this way nature has provided us with a miniature television screen showing the most remote parts of the body, which normally cannot be seen by conventional diagnostic methods, by way of nerve reflex responses.

With Still's disease, iris diagnosis will tell exactly in what organ or organs the lymphatics are deranged. This obviates any guesswork and searching over the body. When we study the lymphatic rosary in the iris it will locate the blocked lymph areas and its channels. Working with children suffering from Still's disease, I personally am very much in favour of using this method, because the children are fascinated and feel involved.

We have to remember that everything contains energy: the air we breathe and the food we eat – our bodies are masses of controlled electromagnetic fields. When malfunctions in these fields occur, such as a trauma or a deficiency, an imbalance may manifest itself in different ways and send different signals. Those signals in the case of Still's disease are most likely to be in the lymphatic system, the neurovascular system or the occipital fibre system, which control all pain responses.

It is interesting to see that with iris diagnosis and Kirlian photography, another aid to diagnosis, one can monitor the progress of the patient very well. In Kirlian photography it is quite clearly shown that the energy passing through a static field is either restricted or increased, causing imbalances in the electrical system of the body. There are many ways to direct this energy flow. It can be done by electromagnetic treatment, acupuncture, or some other ways offered by alternative medicine. With Kirlian photography one can picture the energy field surrounded by living things, detect characteristic alterations and compare them with the progress of different diseases.

One particular young boy comes to mind, who was only four years old when his parents first brought him to me. He was suffering from Still's disease and was quite badly affected. At the beginning of the treatment I did an iridology test to find out where the main disharmony was. He was then put on a sensible diet, similar to the one for rheumatoid arthritis.

This particular little boy's circulation was so poor that it seemed almost trapped from time to time, but simply by administering kelp and a calcium solution to help the blood circulatory system, a tremendous change could be noticed on the Kirlian photographs. The little lad was excited about this as he could see the photographs himself. He obviously did not understand any of it, but it gave him a feeling of involvement in the treatment. His confidence was growing and when I decided to give him some acupuncture treatment he willingly let me do so.

One will always find with arthritic cases that acupuncture is a wonderful help in the patient's treatment. The important factor which I always stress to students is that the correct points need to be found. If the right points are touched, one can immediately see the energy passing in the desired direction and sometimes one can witness some real miracles. However, if the right points are not used, there is no use in treating these patients with acupuncture.

We generally find with Still's disease patients that Knotgrass Complex, Joint Mobility Factors and Urticalcin will bring great relief, and those unfortunate children show such happiness when they are freed from pain. In front of me I have a letter from a mother who writes about her child. She says: 'It is wonderful to see his joints working so much better and he is now fairly free from pain until early evening. For the first time in twelve months I feel hopeful as I see this change in him.'

These sort of letters are most rewarding and make me more determined than ever to help those who suffer these painful afflictions.

Children and adults alike react equally well to herbal or mineral-salt baths and some passive physiotherapy exercises. Warm and hot applications are helpful, and mud, hayseed or sea-salt packs may be used. Any type of sea-salt treatment will have a good effect.

We now move on to a different subject altogether, namely Paget's disease. Again, this is a problem which I am seeing more frequently in my practice. Paget's disease is a slow, progressive bone disorder and can result in gross deformities. It can be extremely unpleasant, especially when people grow older, and can result in severe discomfort. It is found mainly in women. The disease seems to strike in certain countries more frequently than in others and sometimes it is thought to be a viral infection in the pagetic bone. Usually Paget's disease progresses very slowly and in our osteopathic clinic we get patients with problems of the lumbar spine where we dare not give them manipulation treatment. I have seen some very difficult cases where osteopathy was really out of the question in the treatment of this disease.

With this disease we have to ask ourselves if a virus could be involved and, if so, how to treat it with homoeopathic or herbal medicine. I have discovered that good trace elements and minerals seem to be a step in the right direction.

I remember a talk I had with an eminent gynaecologist whose wife was undergoing treatment with me for Paget's disease. He asked me how I could possibly put such value on the necessity of trace elements and minerals in the total biological process of life. Moreover, how could I possibly decide on the correct dosage for people?

I told him that a group of researchers had made the statement that someone with the weight of 150 lbs is composed of:

3lb 12 oz of calcium
1lb 4 oz of phosphorus
2½ oz of sodium
3 oz of potassium
1½ oz of magnesium
1/16 oz of iron
¼ oz of silicon
3½ oz of sulphur

as well as small amounts of iodine, manganese, and far greater amounts of oxygen, hydrogen and nitrogen.

I told this specialist that in my mind this statement was enough to make us think it wise to consider the importance of minerals.

If we were to analyse our diets, we would see that nowadays they are so sterilised and processed that the body does not get the mineral nutritional values it needs. I am sure that Paget's disease stems from an incorrect dietary approach and that the resulting deficiencies could make us prone to attacks of this particular disorder.

My patient was very grateful for the relief she experienced. I manipulated her very gently, prescribed some sun-ray treatment and some homoeopathic and herbal remedies. I was thrilled to receive a letter at a later date inviting me to visit her and her husband. My patient claimed to have benefited so much from the treatment, especially after having to endure such a long spell of enforced inactivity. Her husband told me how much he had enjoyed our discussions and we have now become very good friends. Occasionally, he passes on some medical magazines containing articles in which he thinks I might be interested. I am very pleased with this relationship as I feel it is significant of the importance of alternative and complementary medicine in relation to conventional medicine.

Treatment for patients with Paget's disease could take the form of any one, or a combination of several, of the following therapies:

> acupuncture treatment to relieve the pain;
> a good dietary approach introducing vitamin, mineral and trace elements;
> Symphosan;
> Dead Sea mineral salt therapy;
> gentle exercises, especially after a shower or bath.

Because this particular disease seems to affect people in the older age bracket, patients should try to continue to lead a full life and not dwell on the problem. Try and get some sunshine and avoid anxiety and depression, as these will aggravate pain. Keep interested in life and play an active part in it.

I personally feel that the diapulse treatment is of great help to these patients. I remember the day I opened a Dutch magazine and read an article about this machine, which had just been introduced into Switzerland. The report was very interesting and I was intrigued. I wanted to investigate it further and on my travels with Alfred Vogel I visited this particular centre, where twelve diapulse machines were in operation treating rheumatic patients. When

I talked to the patients, the success they claimed to have experienced was incredible. I then decided to write to the manufacturers in America – and grew even more enthusiastic when I learned more of the background pertaining to this machine.

Clinical and experimental studies conducted over the past 35 years show that many of the effects of high frequency energy are due to electromagnetic effects other than heat. Diapulse was developed to take advantage of this important finding, and to increase the range of application of this valuable new form of therapy.

Diapulse therapy has been shown to be of special advantage as adjunctive therapy in accelerating the normal process of bone and tissue healing, as well as in the treatment of osteomyelitis, bursitis and other rheumatic diseases. Diapulse can therefore be used safely on patients of all ages, without danger of tissue damage due to overheating. There have been no contra-indications with diapulse and it confirms my appreciation of the healing effects of electromagnetic treatments.

If we go back to Paracelsus, who emphasised the prophylactic and healing effects of natural vibrations, we realise that research into nature's own magnetic field has directed conventional medical practice to reform its ideas.

These extra aids open up enormous new

possibilities in the treatment of people where cells or tissue may be influenced by vibrations or frequencies, thus restoring the blood supply to the affected area. We all know that healing only takes place if blood is provided to that area.

Unfortunately, Paget's disease is considered a rather mysterious disorder. It must therefore be stressed that these patients must not give in to despondency, because with the right approach they will improve.

8

Bursitis and Related Disorders

'OH, IT'S ONLY a case of bursitis!' is a common reaction to this disease. In practice we know only too well the problems which can occur due to bursitis and that the pain can linger much longer than expected. A bursar is a small pad of tissue which protects or buffers a tendon as it passes over a bony area. Bursitis is the term given to the condition when this becomes inflamed. If these tendons are damaged, however, tremendous problems can result in connective tissues around the joints.

Most cases of bursitis occur in the shoulder, but other places can be affected just as well; the back of the elbow (miner's elbow); the knee (housemaid's knee); the heel (Achilles heel); deep in the hip (tailors or weaver's bottom); the first joint of the big toe (bunion).

It is usually thought that the cause might range from a trauma, an infection, inflammatory arthritis, rheumatoid arthritis or gout. Acute bursitis can cause tremendous pain, tenderness and limitation of movement. Tendons can be so inflamed that frequently a swelling is visible. Chronic bursitis can follow the same pattern, except that the limitations are often debilitating.

Anti-inflammatory agents are prescribed in an effort to ease this problem and cortisone injections might bring temporary relief. We have frequently experienced in our clinic that disabling adhesions in chronic cases need extremely careful treatment. Manipulations often prove not to be a long-term solution. Generally speaking, one can achieve better results with gentle exercises than with manipulation, which very often is too painful.

Personally, I find that acupuncture, or biomagnetic treatment using zinc and copper magnets, can be very effective, even though frequently criticised by the orthodox medical profession. We ought to recognise, however, the enormous possibilities open to us when acupuncture is used, as this science is thousands of years old.

The aim of acupuncture is not only to release

endorphins and encephalins, which serve as natural painkillers, but primarily to regulate the energy flow using vibrations and energy flow points. With the appropriate use of acupuncture needles, sedation or activation will take place. The equilibrium between the yin and yang forces in the body will establish itself and with proper equilibrium harmony the mind and body will be brought in tune.

Acupuncture is based upon the principle of sufficient and continuous generation and flow of life-energy throughout the body. This force has two polarities which alternate rhythmically every 24 hours, flowing in paths or meridians which are traceable on the surface of the body. On each meridian there are acupuncture points which may be stimulated or sedated by acupuncture needles, thus influencing the appropriate body organs or the nervous system in those affected areas.

The number of treatments necessary to alleviate suffering varies – depending upon the nature of the illness or pain, the duration of the patient's illness or the general state of his or her health. With bursitis cases we have witnessed great results with the use of laser acupuncture treatment applied to the appropriate points.

One of the finest testimonial letters I have ever received was sent to me by a surgeon. When I personally have a statement to make I am always happy to express myself on paper and so in cases where orthodox doctors or specialists acknowledge recognition of alternative treatment, I am more than delighted to receive their written statement.

When I initially saw this surgeon, I knew he was respected in his field and I wondered why such a strong, healthy person should consult me. On closer examination, I could read from his face that he was in great pain. He showed me his arm, which he said he was unable to move. He told me that he had felt such a fool when recently he had been standing in the operating theatre and had not been able to hold a scalpel. He had undergone several kinds of treatment in the hospital, but all to no avail. He desperately needed help and had reached the situation where he really did not care what kind of treatment I gave him as long as it relieved him of the pain. I decided on a concentrated course of treatment and began by giving him acupuncture. The following day he was given diapulse therapy. Later, I also gave him laser acupuncture. He was in such pain that I even saw him late at night, in an effort to enable him to continue with his work.

I was happy with the way he was reacting to the treatment. Meanwhile, I told him that he was eating and drinking all the wrong things, although this had not been the sole reason for his problem. From his letter I quote the following: 'I am very pleased to be in the swim again, as I found the inactivity almost as bad at times as the pain. I wish to thank you most sincerely for all your services and attention, so effective and prompt, and I will never hesitate to come back to you because you appear to be able to offer a wider choice of treatment than we seem to have.'

This was a wonderful statement to make and it shows that the gap between orthodox medicine and alternative medicine is slowly closing.

Arnica Gel, gently rubbed on the affected area, is very helpful when suffering from attacks of bursitis. The rubbing of hot olive-oil into the affected areas will also alleviate the pain.

Great care should always be taken with patients who have soft-tissue injuries, as I have occasionally seen them pass out as a result of the severe pain this causes them. We come across this particularly with tendonitis – inflammation of the tendons – and with tenosynovitis – inflammation of the lining of the tendon sheath. The tendon sheath may become involved as a result of systemic diseases such as rheumatoid arthritis or gout. The tendon sheath involvement may also be due to raised blood cholesterol levels. Strain or excessive exercise may also be at the root of the problem, as is often the case with inflammation in the carpal tunnel in the hand, the hamstring at the back of the leg, or the Achilles tendon at the heel.

In my practice I treat quite a few professional sportsmen, among them footballers, swimmers, dancers and golfers. With such people we come across this problem all too often. Mostly I find that the involved tendons are swollen due to fluid accumulation, which causes localised tenderness. Sometimes, however, the presence of calcium deposits may be visible on X-rays.

One very well-known footballer suffers this painful handicap regularly. Never mind the many goals he has scored for Scotland. I have told him that it is high time he started considering his health and stopped abusing his body, as he repeatedly suffers similar injuries and therefore compounds already existing damage.

I once read an article about him in the paper stating that he had injured himself to such an extent that, according to the surgeon, he would be off the field for a long, long time. His picture beside the article was that of a very disappointed man. Luckily, he returned immediately to the clinic and within three weeks he was able to start playing once more. I later received a card from him after an away match in a qualifying round for the World Cup, where he had scored a goal.

When there are problems with calcium deposits one had to take more vigorous steps. We have seen some good results after homoeopathic injections in combination with enzyme and chelation therapy. This treatment has been especially successful for the so-called 'frozen shoulder'. Nowadays, the frozen shoulder syndrome seems to occur more and more frequently and sometimes people have great problems in getting any movement at all back into their shoulder.

Acupuncture treatment plus gentle exercises can prevent this problem deteriorating and also improve the existing condition.

I remember a famous singer, known the world over, who came to me with this problem. She was due to depart on a world tour and I could clearly see the pain on her face. I used acupuncture and laser treatment on her shoulder and within a few visits she was back on the road to recovery.

Extreme caution should be taken when treating conditions of this kind, as permanent or semi-permanent damage can be caused if the patient is subjected to unsuitable treatment or manipulations. In a later book in this series I will discuss in more detail the danger which exists here.

Kaoline poultices, hot or cold, or poultices made with a fresh cabbage leaf, will usually bring relief. The main aim is to relieve the patient's pain and to restore normal function as quickly as possible. Sometimes I have to use an injection of homoeopathic substances to ease the situation.

From the patient's point of view it is of little or no use to receive the message that a frozen shoulder will get better in time. When they ask how long it will take, they are sometimes told that it might take as long as twelve months to heal. It is very unfair to expect a patient to wait so long. They want faster help – and quite rightly so.

It is possible for an attack of bursitis to settle down after a few weeks. The same is true for epichondylitis – inflammation of the bony prominences on either side of the elbow joint. I have some patients who have been under orthodox treatment for long periods and have found that analgesics rarely bring any lasting results.

In our practice we often have to try and obtain faster results because the patients have already followed the normal channels of treatment before coming to us as a last resort. In many cases, they have already had steroid treatment prescribed by their practitioner. Rigorous movement or forcible manipulation can easily damage the tissue and tendons could easily be ruptured by an injection into the tissue, especially if followed by active, not necessarily forcible movements. The supra spinatus tendon in the shoulder joint is even more vulnerable.

In the early stages of any acute nonparticular rheumatic condition X-ray investigation is most important. I remember the case of an elderly gentleman who came to me with the message that he was diagnosed as suffering from bursitis in his arm. I doubted that this was the correct diagnosis, so arranged to have some X-rays taken. I was shocked to realise that he had been given manipulation treatment, as there were secondaries of cancer present in the upper arm. Even though these particular problems, despite being painful, need not always be complicated, a correct diagnosis is very important so that the resulting treatment may be adapted to suit the individual situation.

The same principle applies to tennis elbows or golf elbows. If the patient's arm hangs loosely at the side, with the palm facing forward and the pain is on the outer side of the joint, we say that the patient is suffering from a 'tennis elbow'. 'Golf elbow' is when the pain is on the opposite side of the elbow, the side nearest the body.

Although I love to manipulate these elbows, and I have learned some marvellous manipulations in the United States, treatment of the elbows is not always straightforward. Pain over these areas radiates down the forearm and can be severe and disabling. In many cases X-rays do not show anything. Tennis or golf elbows may even be caused by a minor disorder of the neck, or dorsal irregularities.

Manipulation (in some cases), acupuncture or laser acupuncture treatment can work wonders for these ailments and hydrotherapy and ice packs can help, but in chronic cases the patient's dietary management should always be looked at. I have treated many cases where the symptoms had been present for weeks, or even months, but in really chronic cases the disease might have existed for years.

I recall a pleasant young gentleman who comes all the way from the north of Scotland for his treatment. He had severe pains on both sides of his elbow. The X-rays did not show anything out of the ordinary. Manipulation was of no use, acupuncture failed and I was nearly at my wits' end to try and help him. A good friend and colleague from the Netherlands then visited me and he remarked on the fact that he had never seen so many people with tennis or golf elbows as he had in the one week he had been working with me in Troon. I pointed out that I had many more patients with similar problems and that they had not all massed together to come for treatment in that particular week. He then suggested to me that I should try giving these patients a supplement of the mineral zinc. He reckoned that there might be a deficiency in common with all these people and he had read of similar cases where a zinc supplement had proved successful.

In the part of the world where I live and work

many people suffer arthritic and rheumatic disorders, which are not only caused by an alkaline/acid imbalance, but also by deficiencies of minerals and trace elements. Surprisingly enough, after he had taken a course of zinc supplement, I was pleased to see that my young friend from the north of Scotland started to react favourably to the acupuncture treatment and the biomagnetic therapy. This shows yet again that patients have to be treated as individuals. The results of basic soil deficiencies may be decreased or increased, depending on that person's dietary intake.

As my clinic is right on the edge of one of the world's most famous golf courses, I have treated many a famous golfer. However, rarely have I had to treat one for a tennis or golf elbow. During the recent open championship I was asked by a famous golfer to treat his elbow problems and it was put right with simple manipulation. He was able to continue to play in the tournament and had every reason to be pleased with his performance.

Again, we realise the privilege of having so many curative methods available to us. Unfortunately, not all of them are recognised by the medical authorities, but the results of some of these treatments are the cause for increased interest. We should always strive for a sensible approach to these disorders which are so debilitating and restricting.

One comparatively new method of treating pain is by a small machine which the patient can safely use at home. This is called TENS – Transcutaneous Electrical Nerve Stimulation. This technique is finding increasing application in pain clinics throughout the word, particularly when used in conjunction with other forms of remedial therapy.

TENS is the application of electro-stimulation on the nerve system for the relief of acute and chronic pain. Professor Wall of University College, London, and Professor Melzack of McGill University, Canada, have worked together on research into the field of pain and through their findings and those of other researchers it has been conclusively proved that the application of electrodes to external points of pain can achieve relatively high rates of success. Common pain – such as migraine headache, neck and shoulder pain, low back pain, sciatica – can be treated effectively by this simple method. The non-invasive nature of TENS and the convenience of patients' self-use (under medical supervision) make it an attractive form of pain relief.

The physiological mechanism of TENS and its techniques in electro-therapy stem from the theories of acupuncture and, indeed, application of the electrodes to the relevant acupuncture points has also been found to be effective in treatment.

It is advisable that this type of apparatus is used

under the directions of a practitioner who can recommend the frequency of treatment and the points where the pads should be placed. As a general guideline, it would probably be necessary to have one 30-minute session daily; obviously if the pain disappears quickly the treatment can be less frequent.

Complaints which may be treated with the TENS technique

Neuralgia	Sciatica
Chronic rheumatism	Paralysis
Headache	Insomnia
Neurosis	High blood pressure
Menstrual difficulties	Low blood pressure
Diabetes	Impotence
Chronic nephritis	Cystitis
Ulcers	Loss of appetite
Constipation	Piles
Bronchitis	Weight gain
Toothache	Weight loss

Stiffness or pain in shoulders or back of the neck

Contra-indications are

TENS should not be used during pregnancy (although TENS has recently been used by some hospitals in tests for pain relief during childbirth).

TENS should not be used if the patient has a heart condition of any type, including the use of a pacemaker.

TENS must not be used on open wounds.

TENS must not be used over the heart or near the eyes.

The old ways of treating bursitis may have been forgotten, but the beneficial properties of hot olive oil compresses or hot castor oil compresses will penetrate the skin in order to relieve pain. The mustard plaster is also just as effective today as it was in the olden days. In my book *Traditional Home and Herbal Remedies* many of these simple forms of treatment are mentioned, some of them more easily acceptable than others.

I was possibly one of the very few people who did not laugh at the old man who proudly declared that he had used some of the finest natural injections in order to cure his tennis elbow. These 'injections' had been obtained by pushing his elbow into an ants' nest!

9

Lupus

WHILE I WAS working in the General Hospital in Colombo, Sri Lanka, I would see many more lupus patients in any one day than I would in Britain. It surprised me that this particular disease should occur so much more frequently there. Over recent years, though, I have unfortunately seen this problem increase in Britain. It is by no means a modern disease, however, because it has been known for a long time.

Lupus is an immune disorder where the patient produces an excess of blood proteins called antibodies and these, directly or indirectly, may cause imbalances in the body. Lupus may be classed as a blood disorder and is referred to as a collagen vascular disease. If the inflammation is not kept under control it may cause permanent damage. I will describe two kinds of lupus, which are altogether different diseases, so great care should be taken to differentiate between them.

Firstly, the Systemic Lupus Erythematosus is the more common disease. The sufferer is very often not even aware of it and does not realise that inflammation is present. It used to be considered as one of the minor diseases, according to our textbooks, but we now see an increase of this problem. Because vital organs such as the kidneys are affected, we have to be aware of what steps may be taken.

Systemic Lupus Erythematosus often occurs as an acute disease which has a lot in common with rheumatoid arthritis but, unlike that disease, it will cause inflammation and damage kidneys, heart, lungs or blood vessels. It is more common in women than in men. Some patients, who have reached the end of the road before trying to get help, finally show scaling patches of varying sizes and the atrophy of skin and scar formation. Even heel lesions often show scars and some parts will remain swollen for life. When this symptom occurs it should be attended to immediately.

Chronic lupus needs a lot of attention. In the first

place we have to take immediate dietary steps. The diet recommended for rheumatoid arthritic patients is again suitable for lupus patients. Equally important for the lupus patient is a cleansing programme. Fasting should be introduced for at least one day per week; also some treatment in the form of Symphosan and quite frequently the enzyme therapy may be needed.

With chronic cases I have had great results with the enzyme therapy using Rheumajecta and Vasolastine injections in combination. The case of one particular chronic patient comes to mind whom I treated quite successfully by introducing a good diet, some fasting, homoeopathic remedies, herbal treatment and some metabolic vitamin therapy to aid the rebuilding of the immune system.

Patients often ask me if I advise the use of sun-ray treatment, but this I consider as one of the worst influences on this disorder, because I have seen many more cases of lupus in the Far East than elsewhere. Any treatment involving sun-rays is frowned upon as it could be the cause of flare-ups. This problem may appear and disappear spasmodically and therefore I would recommend instead that the patient takes a natural antibiotic such as Alfred Vogel's Echinaforce indefinitely to keep this disease at bay.

As allergic reactions are a common side effect of

this condition it is advisable to use the remedy Devil's Claw (*Harpagophytum*). Devil's Claw will treat any general allergy and will especially keep skin inflammations under control.

Another factor to be considered is that lupus can attack hair, nails and joints, and for that reason the use of A.Vogel Urticalcin is often advised, or a combination of calcium/silicium.

Although the disease occurs mainly in the young female adults, I have also seen it in children and males. Therefore it is always important that the correct diagnosis is made and that blood functions and kidney and liver functions are tested thoroughly. These tests have to be done very conscientiously and require a great deal of investigation.

I recall a teenage girl from Jamaica who came to see me. Her diagnosis was that her kidneys and liver were slightly affected and her dilemma was characterised by an over-active immune system. She had been taking some immuno-suppressive drugs with reasonably good results, but had not reacted to any other of the treatments which she had been given, although she had been on excessive doses of steroids. When I first saw this girl I was determined to do everything possible to help her. She was put on a balanced diet and advised to use a vitamin therapy. She drank a full glass of beetroot juice each day and took Petasites. This fortunately brought about a noticeable change and she started to improve quite speedily, considering how long her condition had been static.

When I saw her a few years later I could hardly believe that this was the same girl. Luckily her general health had not been too bad, a contributory factor in helping her to overcome the illness so well.

A lot of research into Systemic Lupus Erythematosus has been done in recent years and some researchers now consider the possibility that lupus might be classed as a viral disease. Others maintain that it stems from a malfunction in the immune system and also there is the suggestion that the cause may be due to nuclear exposure.

I remember one particular lupus patient who had been in circumstances where nuclear radiation might have occurred and conventional medicine had made no inroads on her condition. Neither did I succeed with any of the homoeopathic remedies that I would normally prescribe for lupus patients. An old doctor friend of mine advised her to drink half a glass of the juice of couch-grass roots. In her case this was eventually the answer. After having passed through a crisis with an extremely high temperature, she recovered.

However, I must immediately say here that one of my younger patients, a chronic lupus patient and a dear little thing, is not making much progress with this therapy. She seems to improve temporarily and then, for no obvious reason, she seems to relapse again and suffer more inflammation. After such a relapse she is put on high doses of penicillin and seems to take a long time to make up for these relapses.

I have tried everything I can think of for this young girl and am at present discussing with her parents the possibility of having her teeth checked by a dentist and having any amalgam fillings removed and replaced. Allergic reactions to amalgam fillings can take on so many different forms. I have come across some very strange reactions to these fillings. Even so, it might take a long time to make the connection.

The second type of lupus is called Discoid Lupus Erythematosus. A young girl comes to mind who was diagnosed as suffering from this disease, which is a chronic and recurrent disorder primarily affecting the skin, leaving nasty blotches and scaling plaques. She was very embarrassed about her problem, to the point where she rarely ventured out, other than go to work. She begged me to help her as she herself had already done everything possible. She was lucky in that her doctor agreed for me to take over her treatment.

I tried several homoeopathic remedies which also were of no avail and then I decided to treat her as a patient with a skin disorder. I prescribed Devil's Claw and some sulphur preparations for her and it was interesting to see that she started to improve. While this improvement continued, I told her about the couch-grass method. She asked her husband to help find as many roots of couch-grass as possible, and she would chew these during the day. How happy she was a few months later when all those unsightly scaling patches had disappeared. She was delighted that her hair seemed to be returning to its former glory, as she had suffered enormous problems with her hair and nails, which is sometimes the case with this disorder. She soon regained enough confidence to be seen in public, so her recovery brought about a dramatic change in her life.

It is not always straightforward to accurately diagnose this disease, as it sometimes appears in the form of an erupted skin rash, or it may resemble symptoms of polyarthritis or a kidney condition. Blood and urine tests are necessary to differentiate it as a connective tissue disorder and subsequently to monitor the improvement of lupus patients.

Once the symptoms seem to have cleared, the patient usually becomes very active and mistakenly believes that he or she can forget all about it. It is better that the patient continues with a careful dietary regime. Smoking and drinking should remain out of bounds and acid-forming foods, additives, convenience and processed foods could still have a detrimental influence.

I have also noticed that these patients tend to be more sensitive to stress, fatigue or emotional upsets. Too often I have seen lupus patients who had been treated successfully deteriorate again because of a death in the family or a broken love affair. The original problems reappear, with the symptoms often worse than they were previously. These patients should be sensible and realise that measures have to be taken to keep these unexpected problems under control where possible.

Once again I must warn the lupus patient against excessive sunlight. I feel that this cannot be overstressed. Often the skin eruptions lead the patient to consider sun-rays beneficial to the skin. However, they will have to learn the hard way that sunshine will only aggravate the condition.

As with most diseases, certain patterns seem to be followed. Every cell in our body will change and will have to be replaced every second year. The only exceptions are the cells of the nervous system. If we have serious problems or dysfunctions like those caused by lupus or other arthritis-related diseases, a cell begins to work improperly and abnormal tissue changes will result. We have to recognise what we call pathological malfunctions and that this abnormal tissue change affects the cell tissues or organ, which will eventually die in the process.

We have to do our very best to regenerate the cellular system and this can only be done by starting at the very basics, in other words a good cleansing programme, to be followed by a sensible and balanced diet. Of all the remedies which I use for lupus patients to aid their cell regeneration, I prefer *Petasites officinalis* or Butterbur, a herbal plant which is ideally suited for cell renewal. If we also use a multi-vitamin, mineral and trace elements therapy, we may be assured of favourable results.

Starting with these simple forms of treatment we can arrest any further developments of this disease. Even chronic lupus patients will manage to overcome many of the effects for which Lupus Erythematosus is so infamous.

Because the patient rarely understands this disease, it can be a very lonely road and any literature or advice on this particular disease is always welcome. It will enable the lupus patient to put up a fight to beat the effects of this disorder.

As I have found in practice it is sometimes difficult to use acupuncture with lupus patients for several reasons. I discovered a wonderful method which was introduced to me during a seminar in London many years ago by my friend, Dr Len Allan. The researchers of the Bio Flex Humane Method of

Acupuncture made a good report and I agree with their findings, as I have had very good results with using the Bio Flex equipment.

In order for one to be able to form a picture of the Bio Flex Humane Method of Acupuncture and the associated appliance, one needs to know something of the history of its origins.

In the 1960s, Charles Walter Aufranc, the Swiss inventor of the Bio Flex appliance, learned of the nature of Chinese acupuncture from a medical friend. This doctor had just returned from China, where he had been staying as a member of the Basler Mission.

Charles Walter Aufranc, who had already dedicated himself to the study of bio-geology, was more than fascinated by the subject. He accordingly concerned himself closely with the problems of classical acupuncture and kept a continuous record of experiences in its practical application. While doing this, he noticed particularly what surprisingly good results were obtained, but he also noticed that such results often failed to occur and could even turn out negative. What could be the reason for this?

In order to come closer to an explanation, he felt he needed to understand more about the action of the basic fundamentals of acupuncture. What was the significance of sticking needles into the human body, and what occurred when this was done?

Inspired by a study of the literature arising from well-known research workers, he succeeded in finding the references he was seeking. Thus, amongst others, Prof. Dr D'Arsonval, and the scholar, Prof. Lakhovsky, both in Paris, concerned themselves with the significance of the influence of the surroundings on human beings, influences such as wind and weather, clouds, air pressure, electrical tensions and also the changing fields of force originating from the cosmos. Prof. Sordello Attilly of the San Spirito Hospital in Sassia, Rome, also arrived at a clear understanding concerning living cells and organisms, from the point of view of the material molecule, the atom and the corresponding influence of the whole universe, by means of painstaking studies and experiments. The soundness of these findings was moreover confirmed by the successful treatment of diseases by means of oscillating currents.

Not only by Prof. Dr A'Arsonval, Prof. Lakhovsky and Sordello Attilly were the foregoing results obtained, however, but also by very many other distinguished scientists. The medical doctor, chemist and physicist, Dr Walter Schwarz, for instance, now in practice in Wörishofen, Germany, wrote amongst other things in his welcoming paper to the first colloquium of the 1st International Teaching Research Centre for Total Therapy on 19/20 June

1971: 'I would only remind you, for instance, that every illness has a location factor, is dependent on the climate, and can be influenced by the environmental pollution at the time and by the manifold disturbances in the earth's magnetic and electrical field.'

And further . . .

'The second focal point of our research centre is concerned with man's place in the Cosmos. Man is a component of the Cosmos, inseparably linked, as a Creature, with the Creation. If this link is weakened or completely broken off, illness or death will inevitably occur. *Man receives frequencies coming from the Cosmos* . . .etc.'

Furthermore, Dr Claus Schnorrenberger said amongst other things in his radio lecture in the summer of 1975: 'Acupuncture acts via the stimulation and control of human energies.'

The living cell can be described, then, as a small electrical oscillator and resonator. It consists of a nucleus which floats in a liquid (the protoplasm) and is surrounded by a membrane. The nucleus is composed essentially from tubular tissues of an insulating substance. These in turn contain a saline liquid, which acts as a conductor of electricity. The interwoven tubules within the cell represent true oscillatory circuits, which can be compared in every way with the circuit arrangements, coils and windings of radio receiving apparatus.

The living cell can thus serve for the conveyance or the reception of radio-electrical waves of short wavelength, which in their turn generate electrical currents of very high frequency in the system of conductors of the cell nucleus. The oscillation of such a circuit is maintained by radiation energy. Since man is no 'perpetual motion' machine, however, he must in consequence be provided somehow with some basic energy before his body can convert food itself, for instance, into further energy supplies. Lakhovsky was able to show by means of a series of experiments, that the oscillations of the living cell are supplied with the necessary basic energy through cosmic radiation. In this, however, the continuous changes in density of the field of the cosmic waves have a disturbing effect, changes caused, for instance, by the rotation of the earth in space, and especially also by the disturbing effect of false frequencies which our civilisation produces in the most varied manner: radio and television transmissions, electricity in general, atomic fission of all types, chemistry, including static discharges due to the use of plastics etc. It is certainly easy to see that it is difficult in consequence, for living organisms to maintain the equilibrium of the cells, i.e. to maintain good health, dependent as it is on the proper frequencies. Sickness and suffering would be less likely to descend on the living organisms if the cosmic waves remained constant in strength and frequency, or if man were not continuously exposed to such large disturbing influences. The problem of maintaining health thus depends on preserving the correct frequencies necessary for life, and regulating the field of cosmic waves surrounding each living organism.

It is the purpose of acupuncture to regulate these fundamental energies or radiation sources – which are without question introduced into the human body via more than 1,000 acupuncture points – and to readjust the frequencies where necessary. Reduced to simple and comprehensible terms, this means that when a human cell or group of cells is vibrating in the correct frequency, the cells become or remain healthy, and with them the whole of the organs to which the cells belong. In practice, therefore, frequencies which are too low must be raised (toned up) and frequencies which are too high must be lowered (sedated); in some cases, missing frequencies must be re-established.

In order to effect such changes, however, one needs to know the frequency or vibration which applies at the moment in the case of the cell or group of cells belonging to the organ concerned, so that the acupuncture practitioner is truly in a position to select the needles which appear to him to be the right ones for the treatment: the gold, the silver, the platinum or the steel needles, and to decide *where which* needles are to be inserted, *how deeply* and *for how long*.

It now became clear to Charles Walter Aufranc why acupuncture could be so very successful but could also be less successful or even fail: it is not easy to make the necessary decisions as regards type of needle, depth of insertion and duration of treatment with certainty. It was first really necessary to know exactly, he thought, which exact frequency or vibration was to be aimed at, and where.

He now began, with innumerable experiments, to determine empirically the proper, that is to say, the natural or correct vibration. In doing this, he made the quite definite observation that this natural or correct vibration is exactly the same for all life. If we were able, therefore, the receive and maintain the supply of basic energy from the Cosmos without interference, then human beings in similar states of health would exhibit practically the same frequency or vibration and would live in a state of cell-vibration harmony which would have a strongly positive effect, both physically and psychologically, on our whole life.

After thousands of experiments, Charles Walter Aufranc achieved his object: he found what the vibration had to be for its transmission via the appropriate acupuncture points to have successful results practically every time. A quite specific rectangular impulse of less than 10 Hz, 16 Volt max. and only 5 mA was needed. In control experiments, he found that by diverging from these electronically produced exact values by even a relatively quite small amount, the therapeutic success again became very uncertain.

Charles Walter Aufranc thus succeeded in producing an appliance whose beneficial effects on the health of mankind can hardly be underestimated. The innocuous nature of the Bio Flex appliance should be particularly emphasised.

It transmits the ideal vibration for the correction of false frequencies, irrespective of whether these are too high or too low; if the frequencies are correct, however, there is no further effect. Toxic effects are thus excluded from the start. The current relationships are so slight that even newly born infants can be treated without hesitation.

A specially constructed and also patented pyramid roller guarantees the excellent transmission of the desired frequencies. It is sufficient to pass this roller over the appropriate areas of the body, even if the locations of the acupuncture points to be treated are only approximately known. Thanks to the disposition of the points on the pyramid roller, the right points are effortlessly reached, a so-called surface short-circuit being impossible.

The provision for the attachment of treatment probes for the intensive treatment of individual acupuncture points, including ear acupuncture, or for the re-establishment of missing connections or for the resolution of so-called blockages by the experienced acupuncture practitioner, makes the Bio Flex appliance even more valuable.

Of equal importance are also the Bio Flex 'water electrodes', by means of which the same desired vibration is transmitted and the application of which is especially successful in the treatment of general states of exhaustion, nervous diseases, stomach-intestinal complaints, burns of all kinds, open and badly healing wounds, fevers, and for the regulation of the haemoglobin economy; furthermore, for the support of the treatment of rheumatism, arthritis, arteriosclerosis, etc.

In general, it must be said that the successes from treatment when expertly applied are unbelievably high. Thus, for instance, Dr med. A. Küng in Zurich, in his testimonial dated 11 December 1975, confirms the almost incredible number of 99 positive results out of 100 patients treated with Bio Flex, which is actually identical with the experience of the inventor and his collaborators. The main reason for this certainty of success is undoubtedly a recognition of the correctness of the cell-vibration hypothesis, which made it possible to generate the desired vibrations electronically and to transmit them directly over the illness, often combined with the local treatment of its consequences, results are possible – mostly after moderately short times – which must often, but understandably, sound unbelievable to the outsider. And nevertheless, the whole thing is absolutely genuine and offers the doctor a means which enables him both to economise in medicines and in doing so, to eliminate the possibility of the often harmful side effects.

10

Psoriasis

'I DON'T KNOW how to express my gratitude,' a young businessman said to me one day. 'Just try and think back to the state I was in when I came to you a year ago.' Indeed, he had seemed to be nearly at the end of his tether and had not known where to turn. He was considering resigning from a responsible position because of the big psoriasis patches all over his body. He told me that he was extremely embarrassed to even have to shake hands and had just about given up hope.

As I looked at this young man now that his health problems had been cleared and thought back to what he had looked like twelve months previously, I was again mystified at the way nature works. It has been said before that nature cures while the practitioner treats, and this patient had come to recognise the truth of that. With the help of nature he had been cured – after he had learned to be patient, however. Natural cures do not spring any big surprises on us and patience is an excellent virtue. I never forget Alfred Vogel telling me: 'You have to learn to be more patient than the patient. Nature will take its time, but it will do the job.'

When we consider how many patients nowadays suffer from psoriasis, we should be grateful that although many methods have failed, a natural approach may achieve much to ease this unpleasant affliction.

What is psoriasis and how does it affect people? Psoriasis is a chronic and recurrent disease resulting in itchy inflammation, sometimes with big plaques and silvery scales. Although it is often stated that the cause is unknown, remarkable results have been achieved with dietary management. It is also a well-known fact that it can be linked to disturbances of fats and to the fat-soluble vitamin metabolism. It is equally possible that it is caused by a fungal infection.

Sometimes traumatic experiences may cause the development of typical lesions or irritations and it is characteristic that psoriasis manifests itself in the younger to middle-age generations. It affects both male and female. Very often a family history of psoriasis can be traced.

Psoriatic arthritis, as mentioned in the chapter dealing with that disease, is related to psoriasis. This is the reason that I have deliberately included this section on psoriasis in a book on rheumatic disorders, although this problem is mainly dealt with in books on skin disorders. There is a clear difference between psoriatic arthritis and psoriasis, but as a dietary imbalance can be the cause of the arthritic condition it is most important that the two disorders are mentioned in relation to one another. This way the psoriasis patient will know what may lie ahead.

To begin with, small scale-like patches may appear, which are often ignored. The thought behind this reaction is that if you don't pay attention, they will disappear. However, when the nails or the scalp are involved, the source of the psoriasis must be located as this disorder will often spread to other parts of the body.

I often remind patients that few things are as badly misunderstood as psoriasis. Sometimes the patient is happy with the treatment given at most hospitals. A layer of cortisone or coal-tar ointment does clear the situation temporarily, but it should be understood that the disorder comes from within and therefore needs to be cured from within.

Psoriasis is often ten times worse on the inside than on the outside. Although it is generally thought to be caused by a metabolic disorder or due to an imbalance in the acid/alkaline system, every psoriasis patient should be treated as an individual. It is always possible that other causes have triggered off this disorder.

I recall a young girl who came to me with psoriasis. When no progress had been made after a few months of treatment, I decided to do an iris diagnosis. This is how I discovered a virus lymphatic rosary round the perimeter of the eye. As a result of this I checked the lymphatic glands and noticed considerable toxic deposits in the tissues. I recommended a good cleansing programme to include a period of fasting. I gave her some anti-toxins and also a high dosage of calcium, some kelp preparations and some silicium. This girl started to improve immediately, so much so that after six weeks the psoriasis had cleared almost completely.

This was again an indication that every patient deserves to be treated on his or her own merits, as every case will have its own problem which warrants an individual approach.

Another young lady comes to mind whose psoriasis was clearing up quite nicely with the prescribed treatment. Then her improvement came to a sudden halt. I decided that she should try a course of therapy using Dead Sea mineral salts, available from most good health food shops. The treatment with these medicinal salts lasted approximately 30 days and resulted in complete healing without side effects.

According to results of clinical tests aimed at finding the reason for the accelerated proliferation of psoriasis cells, the benefits of the Dead Sea salt treatment are significant. The same applies to hayflower baths and Austrian mud baths.

I am often asked if a total cure is definitely possible and my answer is that it is only possible if we adhere to what nature teaches us. We are aware of the fact that there may be a genetic disposition which cannot be eliminated with the use of clinical measures. Unless this inherent factor can be suppressed, we may not be able to avoid recurrences of the problem.

What basic conditions are necessary to make the treatment of psoriasis effective? At this stage of the book you will realise that my first recommendation will be a balanced diet. I have been working successfully with the following diet for many years and consider it a good start for any psoriasis treatment.

In this diet for the control of psoriasis a choice can be made from items mentioned under each section.

Breakfast

Compote of stewed apple, dates, blackberries and prunes.

Mixture of dates, apple and blackberries.

Porridge sweetened with molasses or honey and soya milk or prune juice only.

Brown rice and/or barley (cooked) served with soya sauce or stewed apple.

Rye crispbread.

Lunch

Salad of raw vegetables except tomatoes or peppers. Raw apple, grated carrots, onions and garlic, cress and alfalfa seed sprouts are especially good in a salad.

¼–½ lb of grated carrots every day for carotene.

Blended vegetable soup with Plantaforce as stock.

Two slices of rye crispbread or one slice of pumpernickel bread.

Jacket potato, brown rice and/or barley, or millet and potato.

Dinner

Lamb – only once a week.

Beef – only once every 10-14 days.

Fish – once or twice a week.

Take pulses and whole grains for protein requirement – including soya, haricot, aduki and kidney beans, lentils, chickpeas or Tofu – in at least three meals per week.

At least two meals per week should consist of brown rice and vegetables and bean sprouts only.

Potatoes, brown rice, barley, millet or millet and potato.

Pumpkin.

Any fruit, except bananas and oranges.

Beverages

China or Earl Grey tea without milk or sugar.

Herb teas – drink one cup of sage tea per day. Elderflower tea is good or try an infusion of elderflower, peppermint and a sprinkling of hops for flavour.

Drink 1 or 2 cups of fresh carrot juice per day.

Dressings, oils and condiments

Dress salads with Molkosan, olive oil or cider vinegar.

Use garlic frequently in cooking and dressings.

Use only safflower, sunflower or olive oil and then sparingly.

Use ample herbs, especially sage.

Use Herbamare salt.

Foods to be avoided

Chocolate, cheese, eggs, cow's milk, butter, yoghurt, processed foods, white flour, white sugar, cakes, biscuits, bread, citrus fruits, coffee, white flour products, red wine, excess alcohol, malt vinegar, smoked or pickled foods, yeast extracts, animal fats.

Supplements

Soya lecithin and riboflavin (vitamin B2) are especially beneficial.

Also widely used in some therapies is 50,000 i.u. vitamin A daily.

The use of Oil of Evening Primrose is also advisable.

Depending on the individual patient, I may also suggest the diet mentioned in the first chapter. Even after the problem seems to have been solved, I always advise the psoriasis patient to be very careful not to eat pork in any shape or form, citrus fruits, chocolate, white flour and white sugar, and to limit the intake of alcohol, coffee and tea.

The outlines for this diet are the same as those for the other diets mentioned in this book, in that it should consist of lots of fruit and vegetables, rice, nuts, honey, cottage cheese, salads and potatoes. I will always inform psoriasis patients who find some of the medication expensive that I have seen many psoriasis patients completely cleared as a result of a careful diet and by taking the juice of a raw potato first thing every morning. If the potato juice is taken regularly, some evidence should become visible after a few weeks that the patches are clearing up. If the patient also places slices of raw cucumber on the affected parts and drinks plenty of cucumber juice, the skin will improve yet more rapidly.

Psoriasis patients are often advised to eat grapefruit, but personally I prefer grapes or grape juice, which I consider much more beneficial. Cabbage should also be eaten often and in the form of sauerkraut it will be of maximum benefit.

If strict dietary management proves too difficult, the patient should at least make sure that the intake of salt and animal protein is kept to the absolute minimum. In my opinion, when the first signs of psoriasis appear on the body, they should be the first food items to be deleted from the diet.

The second step to be taken in the treatment of psoriasis is the use of herbal remedies. The following remedies are recommended: A.Vogel Viola tricolor and Graphites 6x together with A. Vogel Milk Thistle Complex. The first two remedies are specifically designed for skin disorders while Milk Thistle Complex will aid and strengthen the function of the liver, which is often impaired in cases of psoriasis. If the liver is encouraged to function correctly, the waste material present there will be cleared. The kidneys also need looking after and therefore A.Vogel Solidago Complex should be taken daily with a cup of Golden Grass herbal tea. Berberis is also well suited to the cleansing of the kidneys. Over the years I have seen some badly affected psoriasis patients improve greatly on this treatment. The above remedies are all herbal preparations except Graphites 6x which is classed as a homoeopathic remedy.

Other homoeopathic remedies I would like to mention because of the good results they have all achieved are Kali Arsenicum and Sulphur. The biochemic salts Natrum Muriaticum 6x and Kalium Sulphur 6x have also proven their worth.

All forms of psoriasis will improve when a well-balanced diet and herbal remedies are used. If homoeopathic remedies are used the different kinds of psoriasis have to be taken into account. *Psoriasis annularis*, for example, needs a completely different approach than *Psoriasis palmaris*, which usually affects the palms of the hands and the soles of the feet, and needs mainly external applications. *Psoriasis diffusa* manifests itself in large lesions, and conversely the lesions in *Psoriasis punctate* consist of minute papules. *Psoriasis universalis* is possibly the most common form of this disease and has lesions all over the body.

Using the various homoeopathic preparations we can deal with each kind of psoriasis individually. The endocrine glands, particularly the thyroid gland, may be a causative factor and should always be considered. Therefore a good kelp product is advisable together with some vitamin, mineral and trace element therapy. A good vitamin supplement should contain vitamins A, B and D, a high dosage vitamin C, brewer's yeast, calcium and silicium. This should be used in combination with cod liver oil and Oil of Evening Primrose.

For external treatment I generally use a comfrey ointment. However, other ointments may occasionally be necessary, such as Viola tricolor or an Echinacea ointment as and when individual needs arise.

Another approach to this affliction is acupuncture and the treatment should be according to the acupuncture law of the five elements, following the points which will give an adrenocorticoid action or affect the thyroid and endocrines. Acupuncture can be of immense value as can biomagnetic treatment in certain cases of psoriasis. Copper needles should then be used around the largest patches and treatments should take place at regular intervals. It is interesting to see the scabs disappearing, reasonably quickly. Biomagnetic therapy can actually remove the worst of it at the time of treatment.

Sun-ray therapy is also advisable for psoriasis. Many different ultra-violet treatments are available and a careful choice will have to be made. The only treatment I totally trust is Corona Climate Therapy Psoriasis Unit. Information about this Unit can be found online. This treatment has been developed in Scandinavia and thoroughly tested. The unit is not only comfortable and convenient, but also totally safe. As a result of studies with this ultra-violet unit, it is claimed that of a large number of people treated in this way, 80 per cent of the patients will generally be cleared within six week by having five treatments per week. In Scandinavian countries these instruments are frequently bought for home use.

This sun-ray treatment should only be considered as an additional therapy, to be used in combination with a sensible dietary and medical approach. Nevertheless, there is a tremendous worldwide upsurge in this alternative approach to psoriasis.

Psoriasis is a problem all over the world and it is said that more than 80 million people suffer from this disease. In different parts of Sweden, 39,000 people were tested and it was found that 1.4 per cent of them suffered from psoriasis. Of 11,000 inhabitants of the Faro Islands, 2.85 per cent seemed to be affected, and the figures for the United States of America lie between two and three per cent, or around five million people. In the

British Isles the figure is thought to be as high as one million.

Investigations have shown that in close examinations of approximately 26,000 South American Indians from 95 villages in Bolivia, Ecuador, Peru and Venezuela, not one single case of psoriasis was found and the same can be said for the Australian Aborigine race, only if they continued to live in their natural habitat. Psoriasis is also unusual among the Eskimos and it is said that this is due to their diet and their use of cold-water fish, which is rich in EPA oils.

One report from the 1980s estimated that the average family doctor in the United Kingdom has 225 contacts with patients presenting skin complaints each year. This, of course, included all skin complaints and not only psoriasis. The Alternative Psoriasis Centre in London claimed that over a period of three years they had seen more than 7,000 cases.

In Britain, psoriasis will often be dealt with by the general practitioner, as we only have 513 consultant dermatologists in the country for a population of almost 60 million. Sweden had 6,000 dermatologists with a population of eight million inhabitants and Germany has one dermatologist for every 40,000 inhabitants.

Most psoriasis patients suffer from unsightly and seemingly ever-spreading plaques, which need careful attention. All patients should take plenty of exercise in the fresh air and a lot of sunbathing. Often we see psoriasis patients returning from a holiday in the sun, where they have gone from sunshine into the sea and from the water back into the sun and their patches have disappeared miraculously.

Psoriasis patients who have moved to tropical countries will also notice that their skin clears up as a result of the sun-rays. This also proves that the use of vitamin D, the sun vitamin, may be helpful, but here a certain measure of caution should be taken. I have sometimes seen badly afflicted psoriasis patients who were put on a high dosage of vitamin D, with the result that their liver was slightly affected.

Ladies who use certain cosmetics would be wise to study the formula of their creams carefully as some of these preparations might irritate the skin. Gentlemen are usually advised to wet shave rather than use an electric shaver, due to the sensitivity of the skin. Perfumes may also affect the skin and it is very important to choose the areas where perfumes can be used without irritation to the skin. Soaps and creams should be checked for their perfume content. Jewellery, too, might have an adverse influence on the skin and it might be wiser to ensure that jewellery is never in direct contact with the skin.

I am obviously not in a position to mention washing powders by name, but I have noticed over the years that certain brands have a detrimental effect on psoriasis sufferers. All these external factors should be taken into consideration by patients with psoriasis.

Next, we must of course mention stress, worry and emotion; these are problems which the psoriasis patient should avoid. I realise this is not always possible but it should be attempted, as the greatest enemy of potassium, a mineral in which the psoriasis patient is deficient, is stress. It is therefore extremely important that they learn to relax and try not to worry.

In my book, *Stress and Nervous Disorders*, I have outlined several relaxation exercises, which should be practised regularly, as well as some good breathing training to teach the psoriasis patient to cope with stress. This also applies to women who are affected by premenstrual tension or who are approaching the change of life. I have found that using Oil of Evening Primrose capsules in combination with, specifically, the B2 and B6 vitamin, is always of great help.

Colour therapy used in relaxation exercises, enables us to control our emotions. The colour stimulates the action of the liver and assists purification. I mostly advise the colour yellow to be used, in combination with acupuncture or laser therapy.

One of my patients, a young man, had followed most of the advice I had given him and had even done some sensible fasting. He had kept to his diet, to the letter, and also used the necessary remedies, without many signs of improvement, until I decided to use laser therapy on the acupuncture points. This brought tremendous results. He has had several flare-ups over the years, but when he has calmed down, the disturbed energy flow is easily corrected with further laser therapy. He had always suffered from constipation, and when I used the laser on the points for bowels and kidneys, the external irritations on the skin started to improve. I gave him the remedy Urticalcin together with Molkosan and advised him to dab the affected parts with some St John's Wort oil. He followed this procedure daily and his condition improved to such an extent that we decided to stop the course of injections of formic acid, which he had needed for so long.

Although psoriasis is not contagious and cannot spread from one person to another, it goes without saying that it is advisable to clear up this condition as soon as possible. The longer it is allowed to go unchecked the harder it might become to control.

Sometimes I see that young women improve rapidly when they become pregnant and they, as well as any other patient, should follow a properly balanced diet with a vitamin supplement and also take Urticalcin.

Psoriasis

Over the years I have experienced that nature is the best healer, but psychologically these conditions may be influenced by a positive mind and the realisation that stress and emotional disturbances will not help the problem to disappear. It is my experience therefore, based on the many years of dealing with countless patients and backed up by the many testimonials I have received, that the most important part of the treatment any practitioner can give, is to insist and aim for a co-operative and positive mind.

I quote the profound statement: 'If man can be kept in tune with himself, he will in time be in tune with the universe. He will thus eliminate all suffering and disease.'

Bibliography and Literature

Vogel, Alfred – *The Nature Doctor* (Jubilee edition), Mainstream Publishing, Edinburgh

Horne, Ross – *The Health Revolution* (first edition, 1980), Ross Horne, Avalon Beach, NSW, Australia

Dorothy Hall – *The Natural Health Book*, Thomas Nelson, Melbourne, Victoria, Australia

Leonard J. Allan, neuropath – *Painless Pain Control*

The Merck Manual (14th edition), Merck, Sharp and Dohme Ltd, Hoddesdon, Herts

Dr A. Maurice – 'Nouvelle Etape dans l'Embryoblasto Therapie et les Therapeutiques par Extraits Embryonnaires', *Bulletin d'Organo*

Bibliography and Literature

Therapie, 13 Avenue de Saint Mandre, Paris

Kitty Campion – *Handbook of Herbal Health*, Sphere Books Ltd, 1985, London

Dr Miriam Stoppard – *Fifty Plus, Life Guide*, Dorling Kindersley, London

Sandra Gibbons – *Living with Psoriasis*, Alternative Centre Publications, London

Dr M.K. Polano – *Huidziekten*, Van Holkema en Warendorf, Amsterdam

Paavo O. Airola, ND – *There is a cure for Arthritis*, Parker Publ. Co, West Nyack, New York

Victor Parson, DM, FRCP – *Bone Disease*, Wolfe Medical Publications Ltd, London

Index